MAKING GENDER

Making Gender

*Big Pharma, HPV Vaccine Policy, and
Women's Ontological Decision-Making*

MICHELLE WYNDHAM-WEST

UNIVERSITY OF TORONTO PRESS
Toronto Buffalo London

ISBN 978-1-4875-0920-0 (cloth)   ISBN 978-1-4875-3990-0 (EPUB)
ISBN 978-1-4875-3989-4 (PDF)

Library and Archives Canada Cataloguing in Publication

Title: Making gender : big pharma, HPV vaccine policy, and women's ontological
decision-making / Michelle Wyndham-West.
Names: Wyndham-West, Michelle, author.
Description: Includes bibliographical references and index.
Identifiers: Canadiana (print) 20230216641 | Canadiana (ebook) 2023021679X |
ISBN 9781487509200 (cloth) | ISBN 9781487539900 (EPUB) |
ISBN 9781487539894 (PDF)
Subjects: LCSH: Papillomavirus vaccines – Canada. | LCSH: Vaccination – Canada –
Decision making. | LCSH: Women – Health risk assessment – Canada. | LCSH: Women
college students – Health risk assessment – Canada. | LCSH: Vaccination – Social
aspects – Canada. | LCSH: Mothers and daughters – Canada. | LCSH: Pharmaceutical
industry – Canada. | LCSH: Medical policy – Canada.
Classification: LCC QR189.5.P36 W96 2023 | DDC 616.9/11 – dc23

Cover design: Louise OFarrell
Cover image: iStock.com/kemalbas

We wish to acknowledge the land on which the University of Toronto Press operates. This
land is the traditional territory of the Wendat, the Anishnaabeg, the Haudenosaunee, the
Métis, and the Mississaugas of the Credit First Nation.

This book has been published with the help of a grant from the Federation for the
Humanities and Social Sciences, through the Awards to Scholarly Publications Program,
using funds provided by the Social Sciences and Humanities Research Council of Canada.

University of Toronto Press acknowledges the financial support of the Government of
Canada, the Canada Council for the Arts, and the Ontario Arts Council, an agency of the
Government of Ontario, for its publishing activities.

Canada Council   Conseil des Arts
for the Arts   du Canada

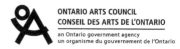

ONTARIO ARTS COUNCIL
CONSEIL DES ARTS DE L'ONTARIO
an Ontario government agency
un organisme du gouvernement de l'Ontario

Funded by the   Financé par le
Government   gouvernement
of Canada   du Canada

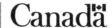

Canadä

Contents

List of Illustrations   vii

Acknowledgments   ix

1 Introduction   3

2 Navigating Controversies and Doing Mothering: Making HPV Vaccine Decisions for One's Daughter   21

3 University-Aged Women's Experiences with HPV Infection and Vaccine Decision-Making   41

4 Media Landscape: Controversies and Competing Narratives   60

5 Vaccine Marketing by Harnessing Hegemonic Cultural Discourses of Risk and Gender   80

6 Gendered Vaccine Policymaking   92

7 Conclusion: Theoretical Contributions and Reassessing Gender-Based Analysis Policymaking   110

Notes   121

References   125

Index   151

Illustrations

Figures

1 Media coverage themes from 2007 through 2016   79
2 Reordering of risk and gender   114
3 Nested decisions to form the frameworks of ontological
   decision-making   115

Tables

1 Canadian HPV vaccine media coverage and story trends,
   2007–16   61
2 Merck Frosst contributions to Canadian medical societies,
   2007–12   99
3 Subsidized HPV vaccine programs across Canada   106

Acknowledgments

I express my sincere gratitude to the OCAD University community for their support while writing, editing, and preparing this book for publication. Particular thanks to Dr. Dori Tunstall and Dr. Ashok Mathur for their encouragement and recognition of the effort and time needed to complete this book.

This book is dedicated to Kyle and Graham, my beloved sons. This book is for your generation, with the hope that in your time you will see more equitable health-care systems and services – a more just world that you both so passionately speak to and work towards.

Edited portions of chapter 2 and a very small portion of chapter 7 appeared in "'What's a Mom to Do?' Negotiating Public Health Literacies through the Traffic between Motherhood and Mothering in School-Based HPV Vaccination Programming," in *Mothering and Literacies*, edited by Amanda B. Richey and Linda Shuford Evans (Toronto: Demeter Press, 2013), pp. 274–92. Edited portions of chapter 3 and a very small portion of chapter 7 appeared in "'It's Really Complicated': Canadian University Women Students Navigate Gendered Risk and Human Papillomavirus (HPV) Vaccine Decision Making," *Health, Risk & Society*, 18 (1–2): 59–76 (2016).

Note: The concept of ontological decision-making, the central focus of chapter 7, has not been previously published and is original to this book.

MAKING GENDER

1 Introduction

Setting the Stage

As I edit this book on the fraught and intensely reported introduction of the human papillomavirus (HPV) vaccine in Canada over a decade ago, we are in the midst of another vaccine controversy – albeit one on a much larger scale. With the arrival of 2023, we have now experienced more than seven waves of the COVID-19 pandemic. Never have we, as a global society, been brought so widely, yet so inequitably, to our knees by a virus. Public health – from international organizations such as the World Health Organization to local, municipal health units in cities across Canada – has focused on ending the pandemic through vaccination. The new COVID-19 vaccines are one of two types: mRNA (for example, Pfizer and Moderna) and adenovirus vector vaccines (for example, AstraZeneca and Johnson & Johnson). The new vaccines from Pfizer, Moderna, and AstraZeneca (initially only provisionally approved by the US Food and Drug Administration and Health Canada) were released into the general population swiftly and with great urgency. All initially required two doses. By the fall of 2021, 73.9 per cent of the eligible population in Ontario had received one dose of a COVID-19 vaccine, while 68.1 per cent had received the two doses considered necessary at the time for sufficient immunity to avoid serious COVID-related illness, hospitalization, or death (Public Health Ontario 2022, 3). Since the fall of 2021, a new variant, Omicron, has emerged as a very serious public health threat due to its highly contagious presentation, although the severity of illness is undetermined, particularly with regards to long COVID (Lopez-Leon et al. 2021). The majority of those infected in South Africa, where Omicron first appeared, were young people. How Omicron may travel through communities of older adults, those with comorbidities, and those with developmental disabilities, as well as the severity of illness for these groups, is yet to be determined (Nealon and Cowling 2022).

Current public health guidelines in Canada recommend a third COVID-19 shot to protect individuals from Omicron-related illness (National Advisory Committee on Immunization [NACI] 2021). Provinces are struggling to get vaccines into arms quickly enough to outpace Omicron (Government of Ontario 2021). It is a race against time, and the fear among health equity advocates is that structurally vulnerable communities will not be able to access vaccines soon enough. Not having a computer at home, having English as a second language, not being able to take time off work, and being far from a vaccination site without adequate mobility are all challenges structurally vulnerable populations face (Persaud et al. 2021). While one has to give governments a bit of leeway, as they are governing "without a playbook," equity frameworks, such as a gender-based analysis plus (GBA+) analysis of public health pandemic measures, are missing from current public health policies. Moreover, public health has had limited success in encouraging those who are vaccine hesitant (Griffith, Marani, and Monkman 2021). A more nuanced communications approach focused on building trust, explaining relative risk, and providing roadmaps for navigating uncertainty regarding emerging medical technologies during an ever-changing pandemic is required. Vaccines alone are not a panacea, and communication from public health officials needs to explain how vaccines work in concert with other low-tech public health interventions – masking, physical distancing, testing, and tracing – in order to stave off mortality and morbidity from long COVID (Lerner, Folkers, and Fauci 2020). The necessity of these low-tech public health measures is not an impossible communications endeavour, but it does require an understanding of how Canadians conceptualize risk, trust, uncertainty, and emerging medical technologies.

The news surrounding COVID-19 vaccines has been confusing and full of contradictory information. Media coverage raises questions regarding which vaccine to take, the availability of vaccines, the spacing and mixing of doses, how many doses will be sufficient considering emerging variants of concern, and the lack of data on short- and long-term potential side effects. This coverage has brought me back to the fieldwork I conducted for this book. Making a vaccine decision quickly in a climate of shifting information highlights how difficult it is to navigate the notions of risk, uncertainty, trust, and, as was the case with the HPV vaccine, gender. COVID-19 vaccines have revealed several gendered variables to be considered when making a vaccine decision, including increased occurrence of side effects and the omission of pregnant and lactating women from initial clinical trials (Beilin 2021). At the time of my first dose in April 2021, the only vaccine on offer in Ontario for my age group was the AstraZeneca vaccine. Pfizer and Moderna were in short supply in the country, so opting for these brands would have meant a wait. Although relieved to have been able to secure a vaccination appointment quickly, my doubts started to mount as news that AstraZeneca presented the risk of potentially life-threatening blood clots (vaccine-induced immune thrombotic thrombocytopenia, or VITT), which are more likely to occur in women than in men, began to surface (Ledford 2021). Being relatively healthy, I calculated that there was more risk in waiting for another brand of the vaccine to become available. I also opted to receive a second dose of AstraZeneca six weeks later; while Pfizer and Moderna were now widely available in Canada by this point, news reports were highlighting that "mixing" vaccines could result in short-term side effects (Reed 2021).

Canada has since stopped purchasing AstraZeneca vaccines. When it became evident in the fall of 2021 that a third dose was necessary to receive protection from Omicron, I was not able to get AstraZeneca. Making the appointment for my third dose was relatively easy, however, as I was on a National Advisory Committee on Immunization (NACI) priority list because of having received two shots of AstraZeneca, as opposed to two doses of Pfizer or Moderna, a mix of the two, or a mix of AstraZeneca and Pfizer or Moderna. Being on a priority list comes with mixed emotions – one is happy to be at the front of the line but also stressed at being deemed "vulnerable" due to a health decision made during a pandemic. To add additional difficulty, I was not sure whether to receive a third dose of Pfizer or Moderna. I scoured the internet, but the news reported that those on priority lists were to receive a dose of whichever vaccine was on hand – as such, there really was no choice to be had. However, when I arrived for my third dose appointment, the attending physician held up two vials and asked, "Pfizer or Moderna?" I froze for a moment. I then had a recollection of seeing an Oxford University study on the success of combining two doses of AstraZeneca with a third dose of Pfizer. Once my shot was over, I quickly searched my phone for the study and was relieved that I had remembered the details correctly.

But my low-lying worry about the potential long-term side effects of the AstraZeneca vaccine has not dissipated, reminding me of how often the mothers and students I interviewed voiced the same concern around the unknown long-term side effects (as outlined in chapters 2 and 3) of the HPV vaccine.

Rationale for the Research and Theoretical Framework

The development of any vaccine is a momentous achievement and a cause for celebration within the scientific community. In 2008, the German virologist Harald zur Hausen was awarded the Nobel Prize in Physiology or Medicine for isolating various HPV strains, identifying them as the cause of several cancers (cervical, anal, vulvar, throat, and mouth), and developing a preventative vaccine against them. Save for the hepatitis B vaccine, which prevents liver cancer, no other such vaccine exists. However, at the same time that zur Hausen was receiving international acclaim for his accomplishments, the pharmaceutical manufacturer Merck Frosst was strategically rolling out its HPV vaccine, Gardasil, by targeting only young women and girls as intended recipients. This marketing approach was quickly adopted by North American governments, and school districts subsequently began to offer the vaccine free of charge to girls in middle school clinics. This marketing and policy approach to vaccination drew the ire of zur Hausen, who spoke publicly of the need for equitable access across genders and throughout the Global North and South (Peres 2010).

Merck Frosst's exploitation of the stereotype of the at-risk young woman/girl and its subsequent take-up in public health policy across North America sparked my interest, leading me to conduct the research that forms the basis of this book. This is certainly not the first time women's bodies have been colonized by corporations or governments, but the packaging of the HPV vaccine appeared to be a particularly complex phenomenon. Yes, the vaccine and subsequent policy were clearly gendered – to such an extent that HPV infection and HPV-related cancer became a "women's issue" in the public sphere (from media accounts to parliamentary debates to television advertisement campaigns) – but this is indeed a vaccine that can prevent the "common cold" of sexually transmitted infections (STIs) and, as a result, a multitude of cancers across gender. How were young women and the parents/guardians of middle school girls navigating messaging that positioned them as vulnerable? Additionally, how were young women and the parents/guardians of middle school girls making decisions regarding a vaccine that garnered much controversy as a relatively new medical technology? As such, how was the fraught proposition of risk – that is, risk that was deployed in a gendered form, both in terms of HPV and the vaccine, but risk that is also very real, as HPV is the most common STI – negotiated on the ground?

Examining women's experiences of navigating HPV vaccine decision-making for themselves and/or their daughters provided the opportunity to explore the plasticity of risk on the ground. The narratives of the women I interviewed involve what Asa Boholm (2003, 158) calls the negotiation of "situated risk." By examining and analysing situated risk, anthropologists are able to move between three points: grand theory relating to risk; individual accounts of risk encounters; and the political, social, historical, and economic context in which these mediations occur. Situated risk allows anthropologists to "problematize structural dimensions" affecting individual risk negotiation and to offer "nuanced ethnographic" renderings of these experiences (Boholm 2003, 158). This goes beyond existing research in other social science fields focusing on risk, which generally zeroes in on either grand theory (see Beck and Willms 2004; Castel 1991; Dean 1999; Ewald 1991; N. Fox 1997; Giddens 1991; Giroux 2010; C. Gordon 1991; Petersen 1997; Rothstein 2006) *or* individual accounts (see Bond et al. 2012; Brown et al. 2013; Crighton et al. 2013; Gross and Shuval 2008; Lear 1995; Russell and Kelly 2011; Spencer 2013; Thing and Ottesen 2013; Tuinstra et al. 1998; Walls et al. 2010; Zinn 2008), but not both. Concentrating solely on grand theory – the metaphysical lens through which the research is conceived, conducted, and analysed – leaves out the important human element of risk, and researching only individual experiences unintentionally reproduces governance strategies. Highlighting individual accounts of risk, without adequate contextualization, reinforces the new public health's concept of "the individual-as-enterprise" (Petersen 1997, 198), a primary tenet of neo-liberalism.

The individual-as-enterprise tenet promotes one's self-regulation through the notion of "healthism," which emphasizes control over one's health and "posits that the individual has choice in preserving his or her physical capacity from the event of disease" (Petersen 1997, 198). The emphasis on self-regulation provides an environment that is ripe for the "privatization of risk" (Lupton 1999a, 5). Nick Fox (1997, 12) discusses how in pre-modern times, the concept of risk did not carry negative connotations but focused on the potentiality of procuring "losses and gains." Today, Fox argues, *risk* "has been co-opted as a term reserved for a negative or undesirable outcome, and as such, is synonymous with the terms *danger* or *hazard*" (12). Francois Ewald (1991, 199) posits that risk "is a category of understanding." Therefore, risk itself is not a loaded concept or event; rather, it is the meaning that is attributed to or affiliated with it in governance strategies that creates the notion of danger or a hazard. In the new public health, risk is deployed as a central theme through "an emphasis on anticipating and preventing the emergence of undesirable events such as illness, abnormality and deviant behaviour" (Petersen 1997, 192–3). Thus, an individual is now signified through a multitude of risk factors. Risk is not conceived of as pertaining to actual events but rather the imminent possibility of such manifestations. Whether it is the insurance industry, which Ewald is writing about, or vaccination policy, governing strategies work to define what is and who is at risk.[1]

How risk is conceptualized and deployed now produces a far more fertile terrain through which to procure and implement prevention programming. In the "individualization of risk" (Dean 1999, 133), if a person does not proactively seek out and enact strategies to prevent risk, it is deemed his or her fault for not working hard enough to mitigate risk. In the case of the HPV vaccine, it is up to women to protect themselves and their daughters regardless of the fact that men also contract and transmit HPV and acquire HPV-related cancers. Situated risk, due to its grounded and contextual approach, avoids these pitfalls. Boholm (2003) describes it best:

> By means of analytical categories and theoretical work, the fluidity and the elusiveness of "risk" as it emerges in real life, in contrast to the abstracted models of ideal states prominent in much risk research, is provided with form and substance, flesh and blood, and human significance. (158)

As salient as the concept of situated risk is to the research at hand, it does not, however, address how gender intersects with risk-related decision-making, nor the specific governance techniques associated with gendered risk-making as outlined in chapters 4, 5, and 6. As Deborah Lupton (1999a, 7–8) observes, "the theorization of risk has tended to neglect the insights offered by contemporary feminist theory and the sociology of the body in understanding the links between gender, embodiment, subjectivity and risk." Sarah Moore (2010, 99) takes this critique one step further by lamenting that, "among all these strands of research – on health inequalities, the medical profession and differences in health care provision across female groups – one aspect of 'classical' feminist work on gender and health was on the wane: the theorization of gender." When risk-oriented literature does indeed address gender, it examines "women" and treats this static category as a pre-given "fact." This academic treatment "has led to the perpetuation of essentialist ideas about sex and gender – the notion that the former directly and naturally entails the latter" (Moore 2010, 100). Examples of such literature still frequent the academic record today (see Crighton et al. 2013; Gross and Shuval 2008).

This book begins to address this theoretical and pragmatic gap. As such, it has been an exercise in examining both situated risk and situated gender[2] through the additional inclusion of theory from Amy Allen

(2008), Judith Butler (2008), Mary Douglas ([1966] 2002, 1992), Lupton (1999a, 1999b), Moore (2010), and Sarah Nettleton (1996, 1997) in order to incorporate a feminist perspective into the analysis. Thus, a theoretical *métissage* tailored to answer each research question is a constant throughout the book. In order to answer the first research question – (1) How did HPV vaccine policy become gendered within the Canadian policy landscape, and how did this in turn lead to gendered public health programming? – Foucault-inspired governmentality approaches to risk (Castel 1991; Giroux 2010; C. Gordon 1991; Lupton and Petersen 1996; Nettleton 1997; Petersen 1997; Rose 2007; Rothstein 2006; Turner 1997), which draw from Michel Foucault's early writings, Douglas's ([1996] 2002, 1992) cultural writings on risk, and Lupton's (1999a, 1999b) more recent work on gender and risk,[3] were employed. To address the second and third research questions – (2) How are women appropriating, hybridizing, or refuting notions of "gender" and "risk" that are deployed in association with the HPV vaccine? and (3) How are their experiences of risk and gender folded into their vaccine decision-making? – late Foucault theory was utilized (see Foucault [1978] 1990, 1987, 1989, 1991, 1997, 1999).

Foucault's writings on governmentality are frequently taken to task for their predetermined nature (Sawicki 1991, 98). Once the spectrum of his writings is examined, however, we see the tightly woven governance strategies of the governmentality period unravel, ever so slightly, in his later work focusing on subjectivities. Foucault, if the full scope of his work is taken into account, acknowledges not only the construction of subjects within the framework of power relations but also the possibility that such subjects are able to level their own limited "critiques," even though enmeshed in the webs of power (Allen 2008, 21). As Allen (2008, 2–3), who also brings a feminist perspective to the conversation, explains, "power works at the intrasubjective level to shape and constitute our very subjectivity, *and* an account of autonomy that captures the constituted subject's capacity for critical reflection and self-transformation, its capacity to be selfconstituting." Importantly, women's narratives provide the intersubjective space where subject formation and realizations/actualizations of the self intersect. It is precisely in this intersubjective space that health negotiation and decision-making occur.

In the intersubjective space, women work towards becoming ethical beings (Foucault 1997). This process involves continually engaging in acts of self-reflexivity or "practices of the self" to achieve one's goals of the good or moral (Butler 2008, 27–8). When referring to being ethical, Foucault (1997, 265) is foundationally speaking of engaging in a relationship with oneself in which we create our own telos, which is our own code or sets of codes for daily life. Scripting one's telos "is nevertheless not something the individual invents by himself. They are patterns that he finds in his culture and which are proposed, suggested and imposed upon him by his culture, his society and his social group" (Foucault 1987, 11).[4] As a result, in the era of new public health, creating one's own telos can function as a form of "self-surveillance" whereby individuals are constantly and actively enacting health measures to keep themselves well and away from anticipated risk (Nettleton 1996, 43). Moore (2010, 103) also notes that "the new paradigm of health is a deeply gendered project, and without such an acknowledgment we forgo an understanding of health promotion as an 'operation of power' that is rooted in gender norms." Therefore, in scripting one's own telos, one is engaging in "ethical agency" (Butler 2008, 28), or what Allen (2008, 2) calls one's ability to be "self-constituting." These actions are, nevertheless, predicated upon normative understandings of gender, even if these understandings can be temporarily destabilized or reordered. The spirit of Caitlin Zaloom's (2004) work has also been threaded throughout my data analysis to answer questions two and three. Zaloom (2004, 368) posits that risk can, indeed, be a productive force vis-à-vis one's sense of self in one's daily experiences; risk is "practiced," a concept akin to Butler's treatment of gender.

Research Questions and Methodological Approaches

In order to provide situated accounts of risk and gender, ethnographic fieldwork occurred over an eighteen-month period and included multiple sites. Research began with three months of archival study to determine how HPV vaccine policy became gendered in Canada at the time of its introduction in 2007 when the virus is gender blind and associated with cancers affecting individuals of all genders (Braun and Phoun 2010). Thus, to answer the first research question – (1) How did the HPV vaccine become gendered within the Canadian policy landscape, and how did this in turn lead to gendered public health programming? – the archival research tracked how the concepts of "gender" and "risk" were deployed in pharmaceutical and policy discourses vis-à-vis the HPV vaccine. This archival research, which was conducted between 2009 and 2010, was then augmented with additional archival research from 2015 to 2017, when HPV policy and programming developments were unfolding across Canada as provinces began to include boys in their school-based HPV vaccine programs. However, I argue throughout the book that the original gendered framework was never untethered in the popular imagination, as is evidenced by a 2016 Society of Obstetricians and

Gynaecologists of Canada (SOGC) advertising campaign for the vaccine geared solely at women. Conducting the archival research meant pouring over documentation, which included Gardasil advertising campaigns, popular media accounts, parliamentary debates, federal and provincial press releases, accounts of advocacy before the federal finance committee, federal regulatory decisions regarding the vaccine, and federal and provincial lobby registries. Critical discourse analysis of these sources revealed that messaging relied upon the overarching notion that women are a "feminine" grouping (Bartky 1990; Moore 2010) – a homogenous and static "whole" that is inherently at risk for ill health, even as medical societies lobbied for gender parity in school-based programs and boys were included alongside girls in school-based vaccination programs. Merck Frosst was the first to deploy this governance technique as a selling mechanism for the vaccine, but if this conceptualization of women and girls had not been in the ether, it would not have been picked up again in the gendered policymaking processes surrounding the vaccine. Thus, the marketing tactics and policy development surrounding the vaccine functioned tautologically as sales/governance strategies.

Thus, the archival research was a critical endeavour in contextualizing women's narratives by tracking the creation and circulation of expert HPV vaccine knowledge and how this information deploys the concepts of gender and risk to enact sales/governance strategies. In tracing this history, I examined what topics were circulating and "who does the speaking, the positions and viewpoints from which they speak, the institutions which prompt people to speak about it and which store and distribute the things that are said" (Foucault [1978] 1990, 11). Tracing this history revealed the *processes* through which risk categories are created and circulated as well as how this crafting creates a risk *product.* In this case, the product is the category of the at-risk girl/woman. Here, the notion of "gender" signifies the homogenous and static rendition of women as perpetually at risk for illness and disease, as circulated in Merck Frosst marketing, and as used in gender-based analysis (GBA) and, more recently, in GBA+. As Moore (2010, 106) explains, "Gender can refer to a set of ideas and images that we recognize as pertaining to, for example, traditional femininity, even if we don't subscribe to the practices those ideas and images entail." As Olena Hankivsky (2012b) also argues, this approach to gender pits men against women, views each as undifferentiated "wholes," and places a primacy on the effects of gender on health.

The archival research provided baseline data on how risk and gender were deployed in these discursive knowledge nodes and formed the basis for interview schedules with women contemplating the vaccine for themselves and/or their daughters. During these interviews, which were conducted in 2009 and 2010, I strove to answer my second and third research questions: (2) How are women appropriating, hybridizing, or refuting notions of "gender" and "risk" that are deployed in association with the HPV vaccine? and (3) How are their experiences of risk and gender folded into their vaccine decision-making? Once research questions two and three were formulated, I set out to find people, places, and spaces where I could conduct my research. In addition to the enthusiastic response I received from fellow mothers regarding the research, the discovery of an additional student cohort to interview was most unexpected.

I was aware of the Merck Frosst campaign targeting university-aged women by the large advertisements hanging in the student centre at York University and the many smaller Gardasil advertisements that were posted outside the campus health clinic and pharmacy as well as in the student centre, but it did not occur to me to interview women students until students of my own, like Sylvana, asked to be interviewed. While talking to my students before, during, and after class, I discovered that campus health clinic physicians were actively promoting the vaccine to women students when they visited clinics, no matter the reason for the visit. Students would often mention that they went into the clinic because of a cold or the flu and would come out with a prescription for the vaccine. Thus, it became clear that students were the targets of a clinical HPV vaccine policy. While not specifically governmental (although clearly a spill over from official provincial policy), similar policies, as research with university students would reveal, were being implemented across the province. I therefore had to reassess how I conceptualized the term "policy." As a result, for the purposes of this book, "policy" is defined not only as "a piece of government legislation ... [but as] a general program or desired state of affairs or, alternatively, as a label to describe outcomes or what governments generally achieve" (Wedel et al. 2005, 35). Unearthing the student cohort was another pivotal point in the fieldwork process, for students brought into relief how prevalent HPV infection actually is.

During these interviews I explored how the concepts of "risk" and "gender" were received, amalgamated, and refuted by women within the context of HPV vaccine decision-making. This entailed interviewing two cohorts of women: mothers negotiating the vaccine for their daughters in a school-based immunization program, and female university students who were the target of HPV vaccine promotion in campus health clinics when male students were not. Interviews focused on how women negotiated the concepts of risk and gender in their daily lives vis-à-vis the vaccine. How did women make sense of and experience these concepts?

What did these concepts mean to them? How did these experiences affect their vaccine decision-making? In answering these questions, I examined the vicissitudes of power – how power was deployed and how it was processed. However, in order to avoid repeating the power techniques used in the sales/governance strategies of the pharmaceutical and governmental discourses surrounding the vaccine – that is, assuming women occupy a static, whole, and homogenous at-risk group – I paid close attention to the nuances, flexibility, and variability that women applied to their mediations of risk and gender in their everyday lives.

Research questions two and three are answered by exploring women's everyday experiences with HPV vaccine decision-making and, in the case of some mothers and students, dealing with past and current HPV infections. It is imperative, though, to define what is meant by "experiences" here. As Joan Scott (1992, 37) states, "what counts as experience is neither self-evident nor straightforward; it is always contested, always therefore political."[5] By "experiences" I am referring to delving into and magnifying subjectivities as they are continually developing. It is important to note that the concept of subjectivities is used in its plural form, denoting multiple incarnations. This book does not seek to make women visible in the sense that *the* missing female voice must be added to the archive (Foucault 1999, 44) or the "anti-archive" (Hughes 2003, 28), even though such an approach would be popular among feminist health activists who overlook difference in order to "provide the basis for a collective feminist subject" (Sawicki 1991, 17). My politics lie elsewhere, in concurrence with Scott (1992, 25), who states that "the project of making experience visible precludes analysis of this system and its historicity; instead it reproduces its terms." I do not want to fall into the very trap that Douglas (1992) describes – that of reinforcing the current social "order."[6]

In carrying out this research, there is the danger of reproducing essentialized notions of gender and risk; researching women only while critiquing GBA and GBA+ as it is deployed in pharmaceutical and governmental discourses that place a primacy on women as a homogenous, static, and universalized at-risk group could be a recipe for certain critical failure. Through the archival research, I trace the social, political, cultural, and economic locations of gendered risk-making related to the HPV vaccine in pharmaceutical and governmental discourses over a ten-year period. This allows me to situate this specific subject formation at a particular point in time. This "historicizing" (Scott 1992, 26) is crucial in establishing the constructedness of gendered risk as a conceptual category. I also seek to unearth how these concepts of risk and gender travel in the social realm between, across, and within different groups of women. If experience is "a subject's history" (Scott 1992, 34), it is important to provide a critical account of these histories. In doing so, however, it is paramount not to "mask ... the necessarily discursive character of these experiences" (Scott 1992, 31). Women hold multiple positionalities through which they develop and rework their sense of self and identity. Race, class, age, sexual orientation, occupation, medical status, and religion are all intersectional positions on the identity continuum (Inhorn 2006). At the same time, however, "it would be wrong to assume in advance that there is a category of 'women' that simply needs to be filled in with various components of race, class, age, ethnicity, and sexuality in order to become complete" (Butler [1990] 2007, 20). This is a tricky line to navigate, and efforts to be mindful of intersectional identity ascriptions guided the fieldwork process. As such, a fluid approach to fieldwork and ethnography was imperative.

The interview component of the fieldwork research focused on gathering women's experiences through their narratives, a long-standing tradition in medical anthropology (see Kleinman 1988). Narrative is ideal for situating analysis in this case because

> texts, textuality, derived from *texto* (Latin, to weave), constitute the locus where bodies discursive and material weave fabrics of the self. The body of each text contains two other bodies which shape the text as it shapes them: the physical body and the body politic whose materiality the physical body symbolically represents. (Smith-Rosenberg 1989, 102)

However, as Butler (2008, 37) notes in talking about her own narrative, narrative snapshots usually begin in the middle, and accounts are "partial, haunted by that for which I can devise no definitive story. I cannot explain exactly why I have emerged in this way, and my efforts at narrative reconstruction are always undergoing revision. There is that in me and of me for which I can give no account." João Biehl, Byron Good, and Arthur Kleinman (2007, 15) also stress that "subjects are themselves unfinished and unfinishable." As a result, there is always a feeling of "incompleteness" (Marcus 2009, 28) when engaging in narrative research and analysis. Thus, I can only claim to capture women while they inhabit the intersubjective space at a specific point in time in their lives. The central objective of the interview questions was to understand how health decisions were made in the intersubjective space.

Interview data was reviewed through a "categorical content" type of narrative analysis. Amia Lieblich, Rivka Tuval-Mashiach, and Tamar Zilber (1998, 13) note that categorical-content narrative analysis can also be referred to as "content analysis" – a process through which "categories of the studied topic are defined, and separate utterances of the text are extracted, classified, and gathered into these categories/groups." I focused more on the data in the narratives than linguistic structures. While this analytical approach may sound rigid, the methodology takes into account the overarching narrative before identifying common themes and categories, which are formed organically from the narratives themselves (Lieblich, Tuval-Mashiach, and Zilber 1998, 112–13). Categorical-content analysis is a technique particularly suited for examining narratives concerning "agency" and "self-mastery" (Lieblich, Tuval-Mashiach, and Zilber 1998, 17). While transcribing interviews I sifted through women's narratives looking for their discussions of the concepts of gender and risk. Once this data was isolated and coded (Shoveller et al. 2010), I looked for the most common themes. When coding, it is important to seek out "recurring, converging and contradictory ideas/codes within the interview data" (Shoveller et al. 2010, 60). I then thematically mapped the data within and between cohorts. Diagrams of this conceptual mapping can be found in chapter 7. Visualizing how each cohort conceptualized, played with, rejected, processed, and appropriated the concepts of gender and risk, along with how they worked through secondary themes such as HPV infection and stigma, "containing" HPV, and pre-cancerous diagnoses, assisted in organizing each data chapter, while pulling all the thematic threads together helped provide an overarching analysis that led to developing a novel health decision-making framework – that of ontological decision-making.

Summary of Chapters

Before recounting my exploration of women's everyday experiences of negotiating situated risk and gender, I offer a brief sketch of the ethnography outlining the chapters to come. In chapter 2, the first substantive chapter after the introduction, I explore mothers' narratives in regard to their vaccine decision-making for their middle school–aged daughters. Mothers exhibited anxiety, enthusiasm, disdain, and uncertainty regarding their HPV vaccine decision-making. Their HPV vaccine decision-making was exasperated by the relatively short period of time they had in which to make a decision and rested within the realm of personal experience – it was not a linear, risk/benefit equation. If a mother had experienced HPV herself, she was likely to have her daughter vaccinated. If a mother was comfortable within the medical realm, she would often view the risks of vaccination as she would another shot, such as the chickenpox vaccine or other routine childhood vaccinations. However, this does not mean that mothers who opted to have their daughters vaccinated were firm that their decision was without any sort of risk. Their uncertainty was agonizing for them. Mothers who distrusted the medical sphere and big business interests were not going to get their daughters vaccinated. For them, the risks of taking a vaccine far outweighed any potentiality of disease. All the mothers interviewed wanted the in-school government vaccination policy to stop gendering the vaccine. Overarchingly, mothers enacted what they deemed the best health care strategies for their daughters, but the pressure they felt – whether it was from pharmaceutical advertisements or public health notices delivered via their local school boards – caused anxiety and a sense of not quite being able to make a decision that they were certain would be the right one in retrospect.

Continuing along the theme of women's response to vaccine decision-making, chapter 3 features women university students' experiences with HPV infection and vaccine decision-making. This chapter is about students' "HPV stories," as one of the interviewees, Sylvana, so eloquently put it. Students called for widespread sexual health education about STIs, and specifically HPV. In interviews, many students off-loaded their anxieties about having contracted an STI and receiving very little social support. Students passionately discussed the gendering of HPV and the HPV vaccine through mass media stories, commercial advertising, and within the governmental realm of current school-based vaccination programming in Ontario. This gendering was so off-putting to students that the majority of those interviewed decided not to get vaccinated or to delay vaccination. In doing so, students resisted the subject formation of the risky, HPV-related girl/woman. However, tautological to this resistance, students were acutely aware of gender imbalances in sexual health negotiation. Therefore, students recounted their challenges in negotiating sexual health where these gender imbalances brought risk into their daily lives, even when they believed themselves to be in a monogamous sexual relationship. Students advocated for more open talk about sex, sexual relations, and STIs. They reasoned that if more people were forthright about sex as a topic of discussion, sexual health negotiation would be more balanced, with both men and women feeling it desirable and socially acceptable to take measures to protect themselves. They were convinced that if sexual education was covered more frequently and in more depth in both primary and secondary schools,[7] not only would young women be aided in negotiating their sexual health, but it also would help lift the STI-related "stigma" (Goffman 1963).

Students were also dealing with the uncertainty the vaccine posed, as it was a relatively new vaccine at the time. With uncertainty, it is difficult to trust. According to Anthony Giddens (1991, 18), to trust in late modernity, particularly in the case of new technical and medical developments, an individual must have a sense of psychological "security." Continually emerging risks work to destabilize this sense of security. If an individual's sense of "basic trust is fragile ... even contemplating a small risk, particularly in relation to a highly cherished aim, may prove intolerable" (Giddens 1991, 182).

The mother and student interviews produced contemplative moments akin to Kathleen Stewart's (2005, 328) concept of a "still life." Not only is a "still life" a moment of reflection, but it is also a creative event. As Stewart (2005, 329) explains, these moments or events hold "a promise that a moment of intensity will emerge." As such, each interview went far beyond discussion of vaccine decision-making. When taking a pause to be interviewed, each woman crafted a narrative that contributed to her continually developing sense of self. As each narrative unfolded, identity was reinscribed and re-enforced, for it was in the thick of the pause that the exterior subject formation of pharmaceutical and governmental discourses and the interior realization/actualization of the self intersected. This pause is what Allen (2008, 17) has termed an "*inter*-subjective (rather than a *non*subjective, whatever that might mean) frame for feminism." Women are not necessarily depicted as "doers," and in the case of HPV infection and vaccine, women are positioned as passive recipients and bearers of disease. As Mariella Pandolfi (2007, 453) discusses, being a "doer" is a term often reserved for men. Inspiration for emphasizing what women "do" also lies with Butler's ([1990] 2007, 22) work, where "doing gender" connotes a continual process of becoming, self-discovery, and reinvention, all within the norms that surround us on a quotidian basis.

In the space of the pause, women are actively, continually, and complexly negotiating their sense of self while attempting to maintain their health vis-à-vis HPV infection and the HPV vaccine. This involves constantly engaging in acts of self-reflexivity or "practices of the self," including actions, habits, movements, and self-framings in pursuit of the goal of the "good" or "moral" (Butler 2008, 27–8). This is what Foucault means when he writes about working towards being an "ethical subject." In working towards becoming an ethical subject, women are creating their own "telos," or set of codes for manoeuvring through daily life (Foucault 1997, 265). Scripting telos is an exercise of invoking power, no matter how momentary, drawn from the social environs. When crafting one's telos, the mothers and students were also engaged in what I term "reordering." This involves the reordering of existing conceptualizations of risk and gender embedded in power structures. Full stop, this is an act of ethical agency. As such, risk and gender coalesce in a "productive"

(Zaloom 2004) manner. Risk and gender were practised when vaccine decision-making occurred. HPV vaccine decision-making is a case study, or a way into understanding how gender and risk were understood and deployed to varying degrees of importance (to answer research question two), and when health decisions were made (to answer research question three). These decisions were linked to the women's senses of self, with conceptualizations of risk and gender differing depending on where a woman was at in her life cycle and her various social roles.

In the next three chapters, I explore the wider contexts within which individual HPV vaccine decision-making was taking place: media coverage of the vaccine, pharmaceutical manufacturer advertising and marketing surrounding the vaccine, and federal and provincial policy-making, which provided the impetus for in-school vaccination programs. This triad establishes how sales/governance strategies are deployed discursively across many power nodes and dispersed so widely throughout society that their "grip" on our conceptualizations of risk and gender is difficult to loosen.

Chapter 4 details national print media discourses and the definitive story arc of the vaccine that developed and predominated for the better part of a decade. The initial media coverage of the vaccine roll-out, beginning in 2007, was negative and contradictory, providing a conflicting information base from which women could source information to assist in HPV vaccine decision-making. Public health authorities and their allies, medical societies, worked very hard to redirect this narrative, but negative stories about potential vaccine risks persisted until 2011, after which the vaccine was normalized in news coverage, then portrayed largely positively. This normalization was further solidified when, in 2015, the *Toronto Star* removed negative HPV vaccine reporting from its record, publicly apologizing for this coverage after an outcry from public health and medical authorities. This dramatic denouement to the almost decade-long story arc points to the narrowing of public discussion forums surrounding the HPV vaccine and the silencing of dissenting narratives in national media coverage.

Chapter 5 explicates how this gendered framing leverages hegemonic cultural logics concerning gender and risk and functions as a sales/governance strategy that places girls/women in a predetermined box removed from sites of power. To keep girls/women in this box, the HPV vaccine is positioned as a cancer-fighting mechanism. This sidesteps HPV as a sexually transmitted infection and proffers a vast platform for sales/governance because cancer, as opposed to STIs, is culturally interpreted as wide-reaching, mysterious, fear-inducing, and multi-causal. It is important to emphasize that GBA and GBA+ as applied in the case study of the HPV vaccine treats gender as pertaining primarily to women. In this rendering, women are translated into an undifferentiated and static grouping of tangible at-risk subjects. While the vaccine is now also offered to boys in school-based programs, I argue that the branding of HPV as a "women's disease" is long-standing and far-reaching, with current marketing campaigns, such as the one from the SOGC, still squarely aimed at women only.

In chapter 6, the gendering of HPV vaccine policymaking is explored through tracing the activities and influences of stakeholders in the policymaking process. The manufacturer, Merck Frosst, took part in direct and indirect lobbying to get the vaccine approved and inserted into programming across the country. The indirect lobbying took the part of leveraging shared interests held with medical societies to legitimize the vaccine. These shared interests, or shared beliefs, dovetailed with gender-based analysis frames in federal policymaking, which rest upon static and homogenous notions of gender and gendered risk. The policymaking would not have been possible, however, if these cultural logics surrounding gender and risk were not already dominant frames in the cultural, social, political, and economic fabric of Canadian society. This chapter provides an overview of current HPV vaccine policy and programming across Canada and highlights the slow adoption of boys into school-based programming and the paucity of policy direction aimed at helping underserviced populations become inoculated against HPV.

In the conclusion (chapter 7), the narratives of the women across the two interview cohorts are tied together through an exploration of the conjunctures and disjunctures of their lived experiences of situated risk and gender. This is where the central thesis of this book is explained in full. The women's narratives indicated that when they engaged in reordering, the concepts of risk and gender were movable ontological modes of being. Reordering involves moving the concepts of risk and gender into either prominence or the background depending upon the context. Thus, narratives from the two cohorts demonstrated that in relation to women's senses of self, risk and gender were elastic concepts. What sales/governance strategies (as explored in detail in chapters 4, 5, and 6) tried to make concrete, women retooled by finding meanings in ways that governance strategies could not predict or control. Narratives also demonstrated that decisions regarding vaccination were ontologically driven.

In closing, the study's findings are reiterated in order to establish the theoretical and pragmatic policy contributions this book makes to the discipline of medical anthropology. The greatest impact this research project has lies in its ethnographic exploration of situated risk *and* gender, and how this research journey has led to the development of the ontological decision-making framework. As Lupton (1999a) and Moore (2010) have so eloquently established, there is little existing research that explores the impact of risk on women and their bodies in a critical fashion. Current risk-oriented research that features women unintentionally reproduces this gender as an undifferentiated grouping that requires intervention because of "feminine" vulnerability. As such, gender norms are reinscribed over and over in existing research. This book attempts to remediate this troubling trend by exploring the nuanced and layered fashion through which women negotiated risk and gender vis-à-vis the HPV vaccine – in fact, reordering these conceptualizations to enact momentary ethical agency.

Women's negotiations revealed complex on-the-ground reordering of gender and risk and the ontological basis for vaccine decision-making. Thus, the knowledge accumulated through situated risk and gender experiences was layered to inform vaccination decisions. These are the circular and nest-like processes of ontological decision-making. As an inherently social and cultural process, ontological decision-making is embedded in women's experiences of finding meaning in their efforts to be good mothers and young women who are made to feel vulnerable in sexual health negotiations, all while negotiating what it means to be strong women as they make their way into adulthood. Throughout these negotiations, women were engaged in generative pauses – moments in which their identities were constantly being reworked and refashioned. What sales/governance strategies tried to fix, women continually unfixed. Thus, the identities women fashioned when reordering risk and gender were directly linked to vaccine uptake outcomes.

2 Navigating Controversies and Doing Mothering: Making HPV Vaccine Decisions for One's Daughter

Introduction: "Still" Moments and Ethical Agency

In 2009, when I began to conduct interviews with mothers of girls who were facing the question of whether or not to have their daughters vaccinated for HPV, the provincial/federal campaign in favour of vaccination was just two years old and aimed exclusively at girls and young women. As a mother of two pre-adolescent boys enrolled at a school offering the vaccination to girls, I was fortunate to have access to mothers in the thick of HPV vaccine decision-making for their daughters.[1] I found mothers in this orbit receptive and very willing to participate in my interviews, taking a pause from their daily lives in order to do so. All twenty women interviewed had daughters in, near, or just past grade 8 and resided in Toronto or its environs. All the women were white and middle-class homeowners who had achieved a minimum of an undergraduate degree.[2] Some were married, some were divorced, and some had never married. There were those who worked full- or part-time outside the home, those who worked full-time in home-based businesses, and those who were raising their children full-time. Their professions included engineers, entrepreneurs, journalists, professors, business executives, and health care professionals. A few mothers had disabilities in the form of mild anxiety disorders. In terms of religious affiliation, women ranged from having none to being faithful Christian church attendees.[3] Most interviews were conducted in person with the mothers around their kitchen tables, in nearby coffee shops, or at their offices. A few interviews were held over the phone because of distance or special circumstances. Additionally, while drafting the interview schedule, I was aware of how my positionality was affecting the questions I asked, how I asked them, and to whom I asked them. My positionality influenced the knowledge produced in this research and my experiences filtered how I gathered and analysed other women's experiences. Throughout my fieldwork I had to work to open up the apertures of my lenses – that of a white, then-married, middle-class academic with two children at home. My experiences, of course, did not necessarily reflect those of the women interviewed, and their histories did not always mirror mine. My narrative and those of the women I interviewed sometimes intertwined and, at other junctures, moved in different directions (Keniston 2004, 233). Having membership in multiple mother and student communities made me a "connected critic" (Bourgeault and MacDonald 2000, 153).

Interviews can be a moment of respite, with this pause being akin to Stewart's (2005, 328) concept of a "still life." Not only is a "still life" a moment of contemplation, but it is also a productive event. As Stewart (2005, 329) explains, being still holds "a promise that a moment of intensity will emerge." In our interviews, intensity surfaced when women reflected on what being a mother meant to them and how this gendered identity specifically intersected with HPV infection and HPV vaccine risk. Mothers ruminated on and processed governmental and pharmaceutical messages about HPV infection and vaccine risk and then accommodated, hybridized, or rejected these messages. For all the women, vaccine decision-making was not a linear, cost-benefit analysis focused on whether benefits outweigh risks but rather one steeped in their experiences as women, including their own previous (and current) HPV infections and what being a good mother meant to them.

Each interview went far beyond discussion of vaccine decision-making. When taking a pause to be interviewed, each woman created a narrative that contributed to her continually developing sense of self. As each narrative developed, identity was reinscribed and re-enforced, for it was in the thick of the pause that the exterior subject formation of pharmaceutical and governmental discourses and the interior realization/ actualization of the self intersected. The pause is what Allen (2008, 17) calls an "*inter*subjective (rather than a *non*subjective, whatever that might mean) frame for feminism."[4] Margaret Lock and Judith Farquhar (2007, 2) utilize the conceptual frame they have termed "living." As these medical anthropologists state, "to make bodies a topic ... is to ask how human life can be and has been constructed, imagined, subjectively known – in short, lived." Whether one places the generative aspects of narratives in a pause, an intersubjective frame, or within the concept of "living," what is important is to emphasize what women are doing in these moments.

Women are not always portrayed as "doers," and in the case of HPV infection and vaccine, women are positioned as passive recipients and bearers of disease. As Pandolfi (2007, 453) discusses, being a "doer" is a term often reserved for men. As a result, it is important to emphasize that the pause of the interview is a space of doing. Inspiration for emphasizing what women do also lies with Butler's (2004) work, where "doing gender" connotes a continual process, not a discrete or concrete bodily motion. She elsewhere elaborates:

> Gender is a complexity whose totality is permanently deferred, never fully what it is at any given juncture in time. An open coalition, then, will affirm identities that are alternately instituted and relinquished according to the purposes at hand; it will be an open assemblage that permits multiple convergences and divergences without obedience to a normative telos of definitional closure. (Butler [1990] 2007, 22)

In the space of the pause, women are actively, continually, and complexly negotiating their sense of self while working to secure their health vis-à-vis HPV infection and the HPV vaccine. This involves constantly engaging in acts of self-reflexivity or "practices of the self," including actions, habits, movements, and self-framings in pursuit of the goal of the "good" or "moral" (Butler 2008, 27–8). This is what Foucault means when he writes about working towards being an "ethical subject."

Here, Foucault (1997, 263) is foundationally speaking of "the kind of relationship you ought to have with yourself, *rapport à soi*." When engaging in this relationship, we are creating our own "telos," or set of codes for manoeuvring through daily life (Foucault 1997, 265). Scripting one's telos is an exercise of invoking power, no matter how fleeting or limited it may be. However, we do not make and remake our codes in a vacuum; when writing one's telos one inevitably draws from the social environs. Within the new public health, individuals are encouraged to actively develop habits and practices centring on self-regulation through "healthy lifestyles" (Nettleton 1996, 44). Butler (2008) expands upon the creation and enactment of micro scripts within the overarching landscape of macro scripts:

> Ethical agency is neither fully determined nor radically free, but is one whose struggle or primary dilemma is to be produced by a world even as one must produce oneself in some way. This struggle with the unchosen conditions of one's life, a struggle – an agency – is made possible, paradoxically, by the persistence of this primary condition of unfreedom. (28)

It is in the negotiation of this unfreedom – immersing oneself in a pause, an intersubjective framework, or by "living" – that ethical agency becomes possible.

A School-Based Vaccination Campaign, HPV Infection Risk-Making, and Mother Making

The first interview took place in September 2009. Carmen (all research participants have been assigned pseudonyms to provide anonymity), who was forty-two at the time, is still vivid in my memory. This poised and self-assured community college professor was clearly a bit rattled, even though she was impeccably dressed in a linen ensemble with a beautiful statement necklace made of polished wood cubes – an outfit befitting the warm autumn days in southern Ontario. Carmen's daughter, Emily, had just entered grade 8, the last year of middle school before high school. Among the forms Emily had brought home on the first day of school was an HPV vaccine consent form. Carmen brought a copy of this form to the interview. It contained a letter to parents, an HPV fact sheet, and required the dual consent of daughter and parent or guardian within four days in order to be eligible for the three-phased shot. The teachers explained the short turnaround as an administrative matter, however, Carmen felt the process was rushed. She elaborated:

> I spent about three hours on the Wednesday night going back and forth saying should we have this done. It's so new. Looking up the side effects, looking up if there were any long-term studies done on it. It seems pretty safe, but everything seems pretty safe when they're trying to make everybody have it done.

At this point in our interview, Carmen paused, the stress of the decision-making process visible on her face. This was a look that I would become familiar with during my interviews. As Andrea, an energetic entrepreneur whom I interviewed some months later, also commented,

> The actual information that came from public health didn't give us a huge amount of time. So I would imagine there were people who delayed that decision because they wanted to do their own research and they wanted to figure it out. I know in some cases people did go and have the vaccine later on that year and paid for it because they just needed more time and they didn't want to have to do it in that environment [the school].

I later looked more closely at the public health documentation Carmen had brought to the interview. The half-page letter was emblazoned with a large logo of the regional public health authority, one also found on building signs, public notices in the newspaper, and posters in community spaces. The endorsement of the vaccine by the provincial government at the top of the letter added to its authoritative tone. The letter began by stating that the Ontario government was providing the vaccination free of charge. The next paragraph – a mere three and a half lines – provided information on HPV. "In 2006," the paragraph states, "there were an estimated 500 cases of cervical cancer with 10 deaths in Ontario."[5] Gardasil (the Merck Frosst vaccine purchased by the Government of Ontario) "can prevent the HPV infections that cause the majority of cervical cancer and genital warts in Canada." The fact sheet emphasized that there were on average 400 deaths a year in Canada due to cervical cancer. The rest of the letter focused on the logistical aspects of getting the three-dose vaccine and in-school vaccination procedures.

The data surrounding HPV and cervical cancer, however, is more complex than was presented in this public health literature. One might conclude that the information provided by Carmen's local public health authority was not balanced, as it did not put cervical cancer deaths in perspective with other cancer-related mortality rates among women, such as breast, colorectal, and lung cancer, which are all much higher.[6] One wonders what purpose the cervical cancer statistics served besides to intimidate parents or guardians.

The fact sheet that accompanied the letter offered six bulleted pieces of information on HPV and the Gardasil vaccine, but there were no answers to any of the following questions: Is it safe? Are there long-term side effects? Does it really work? If so, for how long? The mothers I interviewed sought answers by engaging in active information gathering concerning the vaccine. Carmen explained:

The first thing that I did was go to the ... public health authority website. It was kind of vague and it was sort of "yes" this is great, you should have it done, no problems ... As I started to go through a lot of other websites, it put my mind at ease a little bit knowing that there hadn't been any long-term effects so far and ... it was a very, very small chance of allergic reactions to it as well. That was one thing that I was a bit concerned about because ... my daughter's very healthy. She doesn't even take Tylenol, so I don't know how she would react to a lot of medications. So I was sort of hesitant about putting drugs in her that can't leave [her system].

But Carmen did not gather information solely through an online search. Since the introduction of the vaccination program in Ontario public schools in 2007, there has been a steady stream of media coverage, as discussed in chapter 4. While it was not surprising to see intense news coverage at the onset of the subsidized school-based program, mass media coverage has been ongoing, with a particularly noticeable surge each September as the new school year begins. Carmen elaborated on this:

> At first I thought it was just something to scare people again. When the flu shot became really popular everybody was like, "Oh you have to have a flu shot ..." [and] it's the same thing with this vaccine ... You have a ton of media coverage ... playing on some of the worst fears ... either you getting sick and leaving your children or your ... daughters getting sick.

Carmen continued by exploring different angles mass media stories present:

> When you are reading about it in [an established] newspaper, they come at it from a very scientific point of view. They seem to load you up on certain statistics but leave out other ones, and those other statistics are picked up by these more popular media articles, and they really play on your emotions. So you have the analytical versus the emotional ... they elicit a very different response.

Like the mass media coverage, Merck Frosst's Gardasil advertisement campaign was ubiquitous. During my research I saw it on television, in magazines, in pamphlets in my physician's waiting room, and even on banners strung up in the student centre at the university where I worked. My children even started to point out the advertisements before I spotted them. I was particularly surprised when they pointed out a Gardasil advertisement playing on a Saturday morning while they were watching cartoons. Having had similar experiences, Carmen talked at length about the messaging of the Gardasil advertisements:

> The way they are portraying HPV and cervical cancer, it can happen to you. The people they are using in their ads are everyday looking people ... so it makes it all very real. The statistics that they throw up about how many women will get HPV. Also, how many adults have HPV now and don't even know it. It's sort of terrifying. Then you think, is that me? Did they miss something [when they did my last Pap smear]?

To Carmen, most of the messaging surrounding HPV vaccination promotion, whether through public health documentation, mass media, or Gardasil campaigns, was that "good mothers" (O'Reilly 2004a, 4, 2010) have their daughters vaccinated against HPV; good mothers are responsible for mitigating HPV risk for their daughters by getting their daughters inoculated. The Gardasil advertisements in particular featured a white, attractive, seemingly middle-class mother, casually dressed, with an equally attractive daughter adoringly standing next to her, sometimes leaning up against her mother in a visual show of needing support.[7] Kathy, a lawyer with four children who lives in Toronto, also spoke about her impressions of the Gardasil advertisements:

> I think that the ads are slanted in that they are from the profit perspective, so they are being promoted by the drug companies. They are not being advertised by a nonprofit organization for the benefit of women ... [T]hey are using tactics that make you think that it's a real doctor and a real patient discussing the issue when in fact it's actually the drug company trying to promote their own drug.

The Gardasil campaign has been a major source of information for mothers in Ontario since, as Kathy mentioned, governments and public health authorities have not launched their own public information campaigns. The lack of a non-commercialized information campaign is problematic from a public health perspective.

On-the-Ground Stress: Negotiating the HPV Vaccine for Daughters

The mothers I interviewed were clearly stressed by the short period of time they had to make a decision regarding vaccination. Being bombarded with messaging that tied their decision to the type of mother they were only compounded their stress. Once this stress had been brought up in our interviews, they moved swiftly onto their HPV vaccine decision-making processes and rationales. Of those mothers interviewed, 60 per cent opted to have their daughters vaccinated, while 30 per cent opted out. The remaining 10 per cent of mothers decided to delay the decision to have their daughters vaccinated, secure that if they later decided in favour of vaccination, they could afford to do so. Those mothers who consented had their daughters inoculated either through the school system or by their physicians if their daughters were above the age of thirteen. Vaccination by physician was done at the expense of the parents, either out of pocket or through an insurance plan. Mothers who did not vaccinate chose to opt out because of their concerns regarding "big pharma" and the gendering of the vaccine. That said, placing undue emphasis on decision-making outcomes provides a shallow reading of the data. Decision-making is complex and non-linear and reflects not only a mother's personal health-related experiences but also her mothering strategies.

Opting to Vaccinate: Mitigating Cervical Cancer Risk and Sexual Health Negotiation Challenges

Andrea recounted a decision-making process that reflects narratives common to the other mothers who opted to have their daughters vaccinated. Andrea worried that if her daughter eventually became a mother herself, she might not take the time for regular Pap tests. "Women probably put it off, focusing on their children's health instead," she said. As a way to relay the importance of a woman's health to her daughter, Andrea incorporated her daughter's opinions and views into her decision-making process. "She certainly had input ... We certainly had conversations around what this meant. It was something where – and this is where technology is great – you can go and look at information like this on the internet." Besides talking to her daughter and consulting the internet, Andrea consulted friends and spoke extensively with her family physician. Andrea detailed this process:

> Our paediatrician ... is a highly experienced doctor, and he has three daughters as well. He said that if he ... had to make this decision ... he would 100 per cent go ahead and do this ... it was a hard situation to be in as a parent, having to make that decision, because it wasn't my body that I was making the decision about, but it was more of a preventative discussion.

Central to Andrea's decision was the mitigating of risk for her daughter. As she elaborated,

> It's very similar to things like meningitis vaccinations or chickenpox vaccinations, all of which my children have had because, again, I felt comfortable looking at the risk around vaccination versus the risk of getting the disease or having an illness that could have been prevented or, at least, the impact reduced.

For Carmen, too, the HPV vaccine's potential risks were ever-present: "I'll be very careful watching her [after she gets the HPV vaccine] ... It just puts you on guard." After talking about potential risks, Carmen zeroed in on her rationale for deciding to have her daughter vaccinated:

> This was sort of like a catch-22 because if I do not let her have it, and then if she ends up getting cervical cancer, I'll always blame myself because I had that chance to get her the shot. So that weighed heavily on my mind.

Heather – a physiotherapist and mother of four, with one daughter in grade 8 – also felt there was "always risk with a vaccine," but like Carmen and Andrea, she felt there was a greater risk in not having her daughter vaccinated. However, Heather's rational for vaccination went beyond a "what if" scenario and was layered with her own health history. Having had HPV-related complications in her early twenties informed Heather's decision for her daughter. Heather detailed contracting an HPV infection, which turned into dysplasia some two decades prior:

> Actually after university one of my Pap smears came back as irregular. They told me it was because of HPV and I had to go in and have a biopsy done ... They [the doctors] told me I had pre-cancer ... I was on my own. I'd split up with my boyfriend, I was living by myself, and I was like, "Oh my god, I'm going to die." I remember thinking, "Do I have to tell people [past sexual partners]?"

Heather wished to spare her daughter the same experience, particularly the vulnerability she felt when diagnosed. Heather elaborated on challenges inherent in sexual health negotiation:

> I don't ever want her to go through that, and if it's a way to prevent it then, you know ... You can never trust 100 per cent whoever you are with because they have trusted somebody ... You might even wait until you are married and then, lo and behold, they didn't know and she gets it. She's going to get the shot, everybody should have it.

Both Andrea and Heather spoke of making a decision without their male partners. While they did consult peers, physicians, online health information, and with their daughters, the main responsibility for the vaccination decision fell on their shoulders, even though they both had husbands who were active fathers. Andrea expanded on this:

> I mean certainly my husband was consulted as well, but I guess that I sort of saw it more as a female decision just because I had experienced some of these things that no one else in the house had in terms of having had Pap tests and understanding some of the preventative things that women do that men don't necessarily have to do ... I think mothers tend to do this – we are the ones that take on the role of health management in the house. As a mother, I was aware that this is another role that you take on making decisions for other people.
>   [Among] my friends ... it was seen as more of a women's issue than one that really involved men. So it was not a decision I made in isolation, but it was one where certainly I played more of a role than my husband did.

Heather was even more direct when discussing her role as decision-maker in the household: "If [my husband] didn't agree with it, that would just be too bad. I mean, he does agree because he knows everything that has gone on [with me] … but if he wasn't in agreement, [our daughter] would be getting [the shot] anyway. [*Laughs*] I would overrule that."

Breaking this trend, Carmen's husband actively participated in her information search:

> At first, he said it was up to me. Whatever I decided would be fine. But the more he saw that I was stressing about it, the more he stepped up to talk me through it. He was asking me questions that made me go, "Oh, yeah, I didn't think about that," or, "Oh well that makes sense, so I'll look at this." So, it was more helping me along rather than saying, "You have to do it."

The ultimate decision-making did fall to Carmen, but she received support from her husband throughout the research and decision-making process, which she felt helped ease some of her stress. This was an exception among the mothers interviewed.

Not Vaccinating: Saying "No" to Perceived Health Risks and Big Pharma

Colleen, a neighbour with a home-based business and a daughter approaching grade 8, emphasized that grade 8 girls were being treated like "a case study. It seems like, let's track these girls and see what happens." During our interview, Colleen spoke about how it was her duty to protect her daughter from the dubious interests of big pharma. She was by far the most impassioned of the mothers I interviewed. Colleen was so energized by this topic that when I first arrived at her home, before I had even taken off my coat, she began what was to be the first of many lengthy monologues concerning the vaccine:

> We have a death every seven minutes from heart- and stroke-related disease. And we're spending $300 million, and 300 people a year on average are dying from cervical cancer. Cervical cancer is quite preventable with regular Pap screening. So, what the heck? And this vaccine is only protecting, they say, 70 per cent of the cases. But there are all these other strains of HPV it's not protecting against.
>
> So there's a huge disconnect. So who wins with the vaccinating? … The company that's getting paid hundreds of millions of dollars, and that's just from Canada. The same company is also manufacturing the vaccine for the [United] States, virtually everyone else.

Colleen was not anti-vaccine per se; she, like every other mother interviewed, had had her daughter vaccinated with the routine infant schedule. The common binary in popular and medical discourses between pro- and anti-vaccine (Blume 2006; Jacobson, Targonski, and Poland 2007; Poland and Jacobson 2001; Poland, Jacobson, and Ovsyannikova 2009; Streefland, Chowdry, and Ramos-Jimenex 1999) is simplistic and does not reflect the stances of the mothers and students interviewed here.

Colleen "tiered" vaccines, splitting them into those she deemed mandatory and those she did not. Vaccines that she deemed non-mandatory presented an unnecessary risk to one's health. Our interview was conducted just after the H1N1 vaccination offering in the fall of 2009, and she was quick to point out that no one in her family had had the vaccine. Colleen explained:

> Here's the thing with H1N1 – it's not as necessary. Flu vaccine? It's the flu. The flu mutates constantly ... But they spent all this money ... they were scaring people into injecting themselves and they put adjuvants in the vaccine. And, we don't even know what we are injecting into ourselves half the time.

Colleen's conceptualization of health risk changed after having a child:

> I think that since my daughter has been born, I've gotten much more interested, I've got more invested in my own health. So I'm a little more aware now of [how] what goes into your body is going to affect how you feel. So I try to eat healthy and I try to avoid things that are going to have a negative impact.

Colleen's comments illustrate how she was more vigilant about health risks as she got older and became a mother. However, her rendition of risk and public health literacy was different than that of Carmen, Andrea, and Heather. Colleen's notion of health risk concerned taking in contaminants, such as tobacco, or "unnecessary" vaccines. She also believed that as a society we have become aware of potential risks to the point of paralysis. In response and resistance to living in what she perceived as a "risk society" (Beck and Willms 2004), Colleen chose not to overthink every potential risk. As she explained:

> You never know what is going to happen to you ... I could get in the car – I'm totally jinxing myself – to go to the doctor's, and I might get hit by a truck. I don't mean I'm not going to drive. So, you have to maintain a certain amount of – you don't want to be complacent, but you can only do so much, right? You can only do so much.

For Colleen, pharmaceuticals manufactured by for-profit companies bring about greater risk than the HPV virus itself, and she was actively resisting Gardasil advertising, which, in her own words, was set to make all mothers "afraid" for their daughters. In this line of thinking, Colleen was being a good mother by protecting her daughter from the HPV vaccine, both in terms of the vaccine's potential side effects and the hyped-up messaging of risk, which created stress in itself and was thus unhealthy.

In terms of vaccine decision-making, Colleen, who was married, made all of the health-related decisions in the family for her daughter.

> My husband would not question any decision I made about our daughter's health. Anything to do with this sort of thing, to vaccinate or not to vaccinate, it would be solely my decision – the day-to-day stuff … To someone else it's a big-picture decision. To me, like H1N1, there's no way my daughter is being vaccinated. Her whole class could have been dropping like flies; she still wasn't getting that vaccine in her arm. If they would have said she can't come to school without the vaccine, I would have said, "Fine, you know what? Give me some homework for her and I'll keep her home until this whole thing blows over."

The passion Colleen exhibited about this topic was typical of all of the mothers I interviewed who had decided not to have their daughters vaccinated.

In deciding to forgo vaccinating her daughter, Kathy rationalized her decision by focusing on big pharma. She questioned the $300 million the federal government had allocated to the vaccine effort, saying,

> That is a huge amount of money. So why did they decide to do that? Well there is lobbying and the drug company, so, again, the drug company lobbies, and they think it is a "feel good" policy, and so now we are faced with this decision that you have to make with your grade 8 girl.

Kathy was also concerned that her daughter had expressed dismay at getting the vaccine at school. She elaborates:

> I think there is a stigma around it that still exists – you know, when you are thirteen it is seen as if you have sex a lot. Well, for them that is still a disgusting thing for a girl. So if you get it, it means that you are going to be that way, you are going to be promiscuous, and then there is this whole sort of weirdness about it.

Mothers like Colleen and Kathy were not likely to change their minds as their daughters aged, even if they could afford to pay for their daughters to be vaccinated outside of the subsidized school setting.

The HPV Vaccine and Adolescent Sexuality

While mothers were happy to talk about the vaccine at length, they were more reserved when it came to talking about adolescent sexuality. Even when a daughter was past the grade 8 vaccination age, mothers treated the prospect of sex as a theoretical construct, if they discussed sexual relations at all. Only one mother, Margot, discussed abstinence, although she did not specifically use this term. All the mothers had been teenagers in the 1980s and therefore not generally of the generation to be actively influenced by the abstinence discourse that became enshrined in US public policy in the early 2000s with President George W. Bush (Greslé-Favier 2006).

Instead of focusing on sexuality, Colleen talked about how middle school girls mature faster physically than they do psychologically:

> You see that there are kids in their class ... and the way they were in grade 7 is as [physically] mature as they are going to be ... They have their adult body, they are as tall as they are going to get, they are busty, they are fully developed. But they are still little girls in grade 7.

Most mothers still viewed their daughters as "girls," even though they were either in or fast approaching full-blown puberty. Carmen, however, was a little more practical in this regard and broke the pattern of not wanting to discuss sexual relations with a daughter:

> We are very open about that in that I have talked to her from a very young age about her body, what is happening to her body, as she's getting older. We've discussed preliminary things about sex and she still thinks it's gross. So I'm okay with that ... I guess because I had her when I was younger ... we're closer in age than a lot of mother and daughters are ... So she was asking some pretty frank questions, like why do only girls have to get it. Then someone – a girl in her class – said that only sluts have to get it. I had to explain to her that's absolutely not true.

Even though Carmen was more open about talking about sex with her daughter than the other mothers, she still had some difficulty having these discussions. This is interesting because the university students who were interviewed (and are featured in chapter 3) were quite vocal in wishing that their parents, and society as a whole, had been more open about talking about sex with them.

Sexuality and religion did not enter into my interviews with mothers, except for one lively interview with a devout, evangelical Christian named Margot. Even observant Catholic mothers, such as Carmen, talked about how the Catholic schools they sent their daughters to held information sessions for parents that promoted the vaccine. In 2012, only two of the twenty-nine English-language Catholic school boards in Ontario did not permit HPV vaccination in their member schools (Wilson et al. 2012, 34–6). However, in 2013, Halton Catholic District School Board, which received much press regarding their five-year ban on offering the HPV vaccine to girls, reversed their decision (MacLeod 2013). Carmen's daughter's school held a meeting for parents every fall geared at parents with daughters in grade 7, giving them an entire year to think through their vaccination decisions. Carmen, an active member of the school's parent council, explained the reasoning for this:

> I know there were more strict Catholic parents who were really worried that it would have to lead to discussions about sexuality with their daughters at an age that, maybe, their daughters weren't ready for. Or, maybe, the parents weren't ready for. So our school said the province is recommending that this be done, so we're going to do it. If there are any hard questions, we'll answer them within a Catholic framework, and we'll go from there.

The overwhelming majority of mothers I interviewed – 75 per cent – were observant in their own faith traditions. Ten identified as Catholic, two as United, two as Anglican, and one as a born-again Christian, and they described themselves as regularly taking part in religious activities. However, faith did not come to bear upon their decision-making, save in Margot's case. Margot, a stay-at-home mother of five, would not vaccinate her daughters as she felt it would send the wrong message regarding pre-marital sex. Margot worked hard to shape her household around "Christian values," as she put it. Margot felt strongly that STIs were linked to promiscuity and during our interview quoted Galatians 6:8: "The one who sows to please his sinful nature, from that nature will reap destruction." Margot did not, however, offer the second half of the verse, which reads: "The one who sows to please the Spirit, from the Spirit will reap eternal life." At the end of her interview, Margot mentioned that she had stayed up late the night before in order to gather her thoughts. She was anxious about how her born-again Christianity would be portrayed in my research.

Religious objections to the vaccine and related views of sexual morality had been mentioned in casual conversations with other academics prior to my fieldwork research, yet in the end only one mother raised it as an issue. This was not surprising, as during George W. Bush's tenure as president of the United States, conservative groups did not tend to object to the vaccine. Only when states advocated for mandatory vaccination did conservative groups voice objections, which concerned the compulsory nature of administering the vaccine, not the vaccine itself (Epstein and Huff 2010, 221). The Christian right in Canada has been largely silent regarding the HPV vaccine during its roll-out, and this is, perhaps, as Epstein and Huff (2010) suggest, due to the overall desexualization of HPV in the pharmaceutical promotion of the vaccine.

Doing Mothering

The mothers who were interviewed for this study were greatly stressed by the decision-making that they faced surrounding the HPV vaccine. All mothers, whether they decided to vaccinate their daughters or not, were, in essence, being good mothers. They researched the vaccine extensively and talked with physicians, friends, their daughters, and, in some cases, their spouses in order to come to a decision with which they felt comfortable. In the end, decision-making largely rested within the realm of personal experience. If a mother had experienced HPV herself, she was likely to have her daughter vaccinated. If a mother was comfortable within the medical realm, she would often view the risks of vaccination the same way she would the chickenpox vaccine or other routine childhood scheduled vaccinations. However, this does not mean that mothers who opted to have their daughters vaccinated felt convinced there were no risks; their uncertainty was agonizing for them. Carmen, for instance, worried that there was no research concerning the long-term risks of the vaccine. She felt, however, that if she decided against the vaccine, and her daughter Emily later got cervical cancer, she would never be able to forgive herself. Few mothers who decided to vaccinate had the level of certainty that Colleen possessed. Mothers like Colleen and Kathy, who distrusted the medical sphere and the big business interests of big pharma, were never going to get their daughters vaccinated. For them, the risks of taking a vaccine far outweighed any potentiality of disease. Interestingly, Colleen called me in the fall of 2012, about two-and-half years after our initial interview. She was livid that her daughter's high school sent home a letter from the local public health authority strongly urging that her daughter be vaccinated since she had declined inoculation in grade 8. Colleen felt this was an abuse of authority and would, as she said, "like the state to stay out of her mothering decisions." She, like all of the mothers interviewed, also wanted the government to stop gendering the vaccine. Ultimately, mothers enacted what they deemed the best health care strategies for their daughters.

The pressure – whether it was from pharmaceutical advertisements or public health notices delivered via their local middle and high schools – did not sit well with the mothers. As Carmen pointed out, HPV vaccine–related messaging emphasized that good mothers get their daughters vaccinated. Carmen's engagement reflects the continually negotiated process whereby mothers mediated popularized notions of motherhood while enacting health strategies with which they were comfortable. These health strategies were also mothering strategies. Some may argue that the concepts of gender and mothering have been conflated, but doing mothering is akin to Butler's performing or doing gender. Gender, says Butler ([1990] 2007, 34), "is always a doing, though not a doing by a subject who might be said to preexist the deed." Doing gender is a continual process, not a discrete or concrete bodily motion, as women experienced in doing mothering. Thus, the analysis of HPV vaccine decision-making among mothers traces the creative energy that "erupts" (Stewart 2000, 245) when motherhood and mothering intersect. [8] Adrienne Rich ([1976] 1986) explains the motherhood/mothering dyad:

> I try to distinguish between two meanings of motherhood, one superimposed on the other: the *potential relationship* of any woman to her powers of reproduction and to children; and the *institution*, which aims at ensuring that that potential – and all women – shall remain under male control ... [F]or most of what we know as the "mainstream" of recorded history, motherhood as institution has ghettoized and degraded female potentialities. (13; emphasis in original)

However, Rich's writings on the institutions of motherhood represent one half of her theoretical framework, with the other half reflecting upon the everyday acts of mothering. On the one hand, motherhood comprises the overarching strategies through which women are kept under the thumb of the dominant – and, predominantly patriarchal – order. Order is a key word here. For instance, the notion of the "scientific mother" was created in the first half of the twentieth century when mothers were not considered to be innately qualified to "properly" rear their offspring. During this period, the medical establishment dispensed the requisite knowledge, procedures, and guidelines for raising "healthy" children (Thurer 1994, 225–6). The scientific mother is similar to the "intensive mother" (Hayes 1996) of today. For the intensive mother, resources harnessed in raising children must also be "expert driven" (O'Reilly 2004a, 8). On the other hand, mothering reflects the on-the-ground workings of being a mother – the reordering (and sometimes chaotic and disordering) processes as described and defined by women. While motherhood is a subjugable form of power and, as Diana Ginn (2004, 32) argues, "a form of social control exercised over women as they bear and raise children," mothering can function within spheres of agency – what Foucault calls being ethical, and what Butler deems ethical agency. Evelyn Glenn (1994) emphasizes the agentive aspects of mothering:

> Mothering occurs within specific social contexts that vary in terms of material and cultural resources and constraints. How mothering is conceived, organized, and carried out is not simply determined by these conditions, however. Mothering is constructed through men's and women's actions within specific historical circumstances. Thus agency is central to an understanding of mothering as a social, rather than biological, construct. (3)

When one is able to harness the everyday experiences of mothering on one's own terms, even for a fleeting moment – no matter how covert – the narrative of motherhood can be destabilized. This is evidenced in the narratives of the women interviewed, which harnessed the good mother discourse by enacting intensive mothering to productive effect. This is not, however, "authentic mothering" (O'Reilly 2004b, 10), a term that inadvertently reifies mothering by bringing forth a singular mothering model against which mothers can be judged.

When motherhood and mothering intersected, mothers strategically accommodated, rejected, and hybridized the institutional directives that were embedded in HPV vaccine public health, mass media, and pharmaceutical messaging, thus engaging in a reordering of dominant HPV vaccine–related discourses. While women initially appeared to echo dominant discourses surrounding motherhood, a closer examination revealed how they were refashioning the good mother precept in novel ways. Engaging in reordering while making a vaccine decision for a daughter provided the women with the opportunity to reproduce, recreate, and re-enforce an aspect of their own sense of self: their sense of being a mother.[9]

The active negotiation of being a good mother resulted in different vaccine mediation strategies. Rationales varied, furthermore, among those who made similar decisions – whether opting in favour of or against vaccination or delaying that decision. For example, while both Andrea and Heather decided to have their daughters vaccinated, Heather's experience of HPV-related complications in her early twenties primarily informed her decision for her daughter. Andrea provided a salient example of formulating health strategies linked to the very conceptualization of mothering that, instead of being contradictory, was steeped in irony. As Butler (2004, 3) states, "[the fact] that my agency is riven with paradox does not mean it is impossible. It only means that paradox is the condition of its possibility." Andrea sought to shield her daughter from the downsides of intensive mothering someday, all the while clearly enacting these tenets herself. Andrea's vaccine decision may have mirrored dominant motherhood discourses, but she was, momentarily, attempting to disrupt future hegemonic conceptualizations of motherhood so that her daughter would not have to do the same when she grew up. Thus, to form her own mothering strategies within the context of vaccine decision-making and doing mothering was an act of hope. Just because she had to navigate the maze of motherhood did not mean that her daughter should have to negotiate these same ideological frameworks. While Andrea's creative mothering strategies will not dismantle the overarching structures of motherhood, she began to loosen their grip. Her approach was a move to "undo restrictively normative conceptions of sexual and gendered life" (Butler 2004, 1).

Neither Andrea nor Heather felt that the vaccine posed undue risk to their daughters. Andrea believed that the vaccine was similar in terms of risk to other childhood vaccines for meningitis or chickenpox. While Heather, too, believed that all vaccines are potentially risky, her own difficult experience with HPV and related interventions outweighed concerns of risk related to the HPV vaccine.

Among those mothers who decided against vaccination, the recrafting of these same discourses took a different turn. These mothers refashioned the popularized conceptualization of the good mother to stand for mothers who did extensive research regarding the effects of the HPV vaccine, did not want their daughters to be "test" subjects for a vaccine that had not been on the market for very long, and who cared enough to say "no." These mothers, Colleen being one, reinforced how pervasive the good mother and intensive mothering discourses are, regardless of a vaccination decision. In response and resistance to living in what she conceived of as a "risk society," Colleen chose not to overthink every potential risk. Thus, for Colleen, pharmaceuticals, which are manufactured by for-profit companies, brought about greater risk than the HPV virus itself, and she actively resisted Gardasil advertising that, in her own words, was set to make all mothers "afraid" for their daughters. For Andrea, Heather, and Colleen, HPV infection risk was also a far-off proposition; their daughters were not yet sexually active (at least to their knowledge). For those who opted for vaccination, long-term vaccine side effects were years away from materializing, if they developed at all. Thus, despite their differing mothering strategies, both the mothers who had their daughters vaccinated and those who did not considered HPV infection and HPV vaccine–related risk a far off possibility.

Conclusion

The mothers who were interviewed for this study were greatly stressed by the decision-making that they faced surrounding the HPV vaccine. As Carmen stated, "it weighs heavily on my mind." All mothers, whether they decided to vaccinate or not, were, in essence, being good mothers. They researched the vaccine extensively and talked with physicians, friends, and their daughters in order to come to a decision with which they felt comfortable. In the end, decision-making rested within the realm of personal experience – it was not a linear, risk/benefit equation. If a mother, like Heather, had experienced HPV herself, she was likely to have her daughter vaccinated. If a mother was comfortable within the medical realm, she would often view the risks of vaccination as she would another shot, such as the chickenpox vaccine or other routine childhood scheduled vaccinations. This does not mean, however, that mothers who opted to have their daughters vaccinated were firmly convinced that their decision was without any sort of risk. Their uncertainty was agonizing for them. For example, Carmen felt she was potentially bringing risk to her daughter Emily because there was no body of research concerning the long-term risks of the vaccine. However, if she did not get Emily vaccinated, and Emily did eventually get cervical cancer, Carmen would never forgive herself. Few mothers who decided to vaccinate had the level of certainty that Colleen possessed. Mothers like Colleen and Kathy, who distrusted the medical sphere and big business interests, such as big pharma, were never going to get their daughters vaccinated. For them, the risks of taking a vaccine far outweighed any potentiality of disease. Colleen also later voiced how she would "like the state to stay out of her mothering decisions," and all of the mothers interviewed wanted the in-school government vaccination policy to stop gendering the vaccine.

Ultimately, mothers enacted what they deemed the best health care strategies for their daughters, but the pressure to vaccinate – whether it was stemming from pharmaceutical advertisements or public health notices delivered via their the local high schools – did not sit well with them. When reordering risk and gender, mothers were actively "doing" mothering – weaving nets of experience, which, when assembled, helped form their ethical being or sense of self. For example, mothers were deeply entrenched in performing their versions of being a good mother. This encompassed navigating the opposing spheres of motherhood and mothering and finding a comfortable space for themselves somewhere in between these two ideological and pragmatic constructs. This navigation was made possible by enacting numerous forms of intensive mothering, wherein mothers "do" plenty. They researched vaccines, consulted widely about their daughters' health, and actively participated in mothering so that, ironically, their daughters would not have to be so "hands-on" when they became mothers themselves.

3 University-Aged Women's Experiences with HPV Infection and Vaccine Decision-Making

Introduction

This chapter is about university students' "HPV stories," as Sylvana so eloquently put it. It is about their urging for widespread sexual health education concerning STIs, specifically HPV, and their deliberations surrounding the HPV vaccine. Interviews were intense and emotion-filled events in which students off-loaded their anxieties about having contracted an STI, genital warts, or cervical dysplasia and receiving very little social support. Many felt too stigmatized to share their experiences with friends, family, and peers. These experiences led students to strongly urge for in-school and public health-oriented sexual health education programming, which could help destigmatize STIs and bring an element of balance between partners into sexual health negotiation. Young women are too often tasked with the responsibility of ensuring "safe" sexual health negotiation within sexual encounters and bear the brunt of the blame when an STI is contracted. Being positioned as bearers of sexual disease (as is demonstrated and reinforced in HPV vaccine advertising and the fact that school vaccination programs were aimed only at girls for a decade) leaves them feeling vulnerable. The gendering of HPV and the HPV vaccine, both through Merck Frosst marketing and within the governmental realm of school-based vaccination programming in Ontario combined with uncertainty vis-à-vis potential long-term side effects meant that the majority of students interviewed decided not to get vaccinated or to delay vaccination. Their saying "no" to the vaccine was their way of saying "no" to HPV gendering and potential vaccine risks.

All twenty-four students interviewed were in the process of earning undergraduate, graduate, or professional degrees. Areas of specialization varied from women's studies to law to kinesiology. I did notice that many students were in health-related fields, particularly nursing. In terms of age, students ranged from their early to late twenties. Just under half of the students were in heterosexual relationships, engaged, or married. Despite efforts to recruit non-heterosexual students, I was not successful in this regard. I did send out a call for participants to an LGBTQ2+ student group, but despite the group director's enthusiasm for my project, I did not receive any responses through this recruitment avenue. However, this cohort of interviewees was slightly more ethnically diverse than the mothers, with a handful self-describing as being of Asian or Afro-Caribbean descent.

HPV Stories: Genital Wart and Cervical Dysplasia Experiences

One cold afternoon, Sylvana entered my office, took off her large, puffy winter coat, and sat on the chair set out for her. She had with her a large knapsack-cum-suitcase, which she opened to reveal several file folders of HPV research. Evidently, Sylvana had thoroughly prepared for our interview, which was not surprising, considering she was a health sciences major. After bringing out her research, Sylvana sat down, sighed loudly, and asked how I was doing. After formal pleasantries were exchanged, Sylvana delved straight into her HPV story:

> I was scheduled for a specialist appointment because I have a few enlarged lymph nodes. I have the practice of getting all of my medical results together every time I see a specialist and just presenting them to the specialists just in case, you know, they can make sense of something that I can't tell them.
>   Among the results there was this piece of paper that said *Condyloma acuminata* [genital warts] on it, and I was like, "Oh, I don't remember this one." So I read through it and it turns out it was the histopathological report from when I went to see the dermatologist in the spring for what they call a "skin tag." Both my family doctor and the dermatologist thought that it was just a vulvarous skin tag, but it turned out it was *Condyloma acuminata*, which is caused by HPV. I was shocked.

Not only was Sylvana startled to find out she had genital warts – without notice from a physician or the physician's office – but she was also surprised that such a lapse in information sharing occurred in Canada, as she felt she had received excellent care here, as opposed to her experience in her native Slovakia. Sylvana explained how she reacted to the unexpected news and her subsequent course of action:

> I called the dermatologist's office and then when I saw the doctor I said, "How come nobody called me about this?" She said, "Well I did write down

for the secretary to call you and nobody called you?" I said, "No." *Condyloma acuminata* is a big deal, but it is not as big of a deal as finding out that you have cancer by yourself or something worse.

Maya, a twenty-seven-year-old master of nursing student researching sexual health education, had a similar story. She described her experiences contracting herpes and genital warts:

> I had herpes when I was nineteen ... That virus is very complex ... and I think it's so weird because of the very, very serious association between depression and herpes. No one really has ever thought about that, right? They think, okay, it's an STI, you get it, but there's so much, so many layers of psychosocial stigma attached to it. I'm sure the same thing can be said for HPV ... there's so much emotionally that goes on with women. And that's not being talked about and it's not being part of our treatment that we get when we have this. We're not given the support that's really necessary in order to cope with this.

A culmination of personal experience and academic training led Maya to passionately advocate for a social reframing of STIs. Instead of being considered a big or traumatic event, she argued that "people should think of HPV as part of a normal, healthy sexuality, because it can't necessarily be prevented, so if you are going to have sex, you are going to end of up getting HPV ... and it will go away on its own for the most part. The stigma is so silly because everyone is going to have it at some point."

While Maya was very pragmatic about STIs, Sylvana was not as relaxed and needed some time to get over the initial shock of her discovery. Additionally, Sylvana was worried about the long-term implications of having contracted genital warts. She talked about her fears regarding the impact that an HPV infection today could have on any future children she might have:

> My first thought was, "How is that going to influence the fact that I want to become a mother one day?" Because it's extremely rare, but my understanding is that in some cases children can get laryngeal warts while in utero, and there are other effects that a woman's infection can have on the child. So I was really scared ... to me, that would be extremely humiliating to have my – I guess I could call it [my] irresponsibility of not wearing a condom, stamped on my child's body.

Sylvana did not just want to ruminate about the potential future effects of an HPV infection but also needed to share her current experiences:

I am clear of it now, but my boyfriend is just on his last treatment. I've been researching non-stop. Thank god mine aren't internal … they are just on the outside of the surface of the skin and … like they said, that's a low, low type of HPV …[1]

My boyfriend, he didn't have any on the head of his penis. I was thankful for that because it would have put me into more complications, more problems. I don't even know what the treatment would have been, because that area is so sensitive.

Sylvana explained that she and her boyfriend did not even realize they had genital warts until her discovery while leafing through her medical records. As we spoke in my office on that cold Toronto winter day, I was beginning to understand why Sylvana so urgently wanted to talk to me. She had been holding in a lot regarding her HPV infection.

Madeleine, an undergraduate liberal arts major, was also eager to share her HPV story with me – so much so, that we had our interview over the phone while she was skating on the Rideau Canal in Ottawa on a frigid February morning. Madeleine had experienced cervical dysplasia but not genital warts. Madeleine explains:

I didn't have any symptoms, you know. There was nothing going on with me; I had no idea. It was really scary, and you think you have cancer. That was the biggest misconception. You can take a biopsy initially when the HPV is found and … the first thing they say is you don't have cancer, and that's really relieving, because when you think HPV, you think automatically, "I have cervical cancer."

Having received abnormal Pap test results for two and a half years, indicating that her body would not likely clear the infection on its own, Madeleine underwent a loop electrosurgical excision procedure (LEEP) at a hospital colposcopy clinic. Madeleine was very appreciative of the care she received there. And unlike Sylvana, who exhibited discomfort while talking about genital warts, Madeleine was very open about her cervical dysplasia with her peers, emphasizing that she was helping a friend prepare for her upcoming LEEP and that among her peer group HPV infection was common. While Madeleine was comfortable talking about sex and had a strong grasp of HPV etiology, she, like other students, such as Sylvana and Maya, advocated for expanded sexual health education surrounding HPV for young women who are not so at ease discussing sex.

Talking about Sex: HPV Infection and Sexual Health Negotiation

Sylvana was, understandably, concerned about how she got a genital wart infection.[2] She felt that having had only a few sexual partners helped narrow down the source.

> My previous sexual partners were all virgins,[3] so I knew it was very easy for me to bring it down from whom I had it, right? So it was clearly from my [current] boyfriend, and I talked to him about it, and I told him clearly that it was from him. That being said, I don't know if my sexual practices have changed because there is not much that you can change in relation to this diagnosis.

When speaking about getting HPV from her boyfriend, Sylvana brought her narrative to the issue of relationship fidelity, a concern for many students because it exposes how vulnerable their sexual health is. Sylvana gave her perspective:

> I think that the first step to preventing them [genital warts] is communication between partners and equal involvement of both partners in awareness of their risks and just check-ups and things like that, like knowing your status related to various diseases and knowing your risks and communicating with your partner. So, I think that even though the medical institutions are trying so hard to detect it [HPV transmission] and prevent it, regardless of how hard they try, if there is no communication at the couple level, then all of the attempts are just futile.

When there is a breakdown in communication, as Sylvana put it, women are left exposed. At the time of our interview, Sylvana was undecided as to whether or not she would get the HPV vaccine. Her decision hinged upon fidelity:

> I think it boils down to my relationship with my partner, which is really weird because it definitely shouldn't be like that. I should just really think of just getting it. In the end, people are just, their natural approach is to just give in to trusting the other and hope to just really have a monogamous relationship, at least most girls would want that probably – most girls, I would say. Probably in the next two years if I find that I can rebuild my confidence in my partner, then probably I won't get it, but if not, then I guess I'll get it. So in the end it just depends on my relationship rather than any other factor.

Sylvana's call for more open communication surrounding sex – whether between partners, among peers, or within popular discourse – was a common sentiment expressed by students. It is precisely such open communication that was lacking in the Ontario government's school-based HPV vaccination program, according to Sylvana. She remarked how an HPV educational campaign was markedly absent from this public health initiative. According to her, a shift in strategy is required:

> The government should really focus on giving people enough education on sexual communication ... while people are in school ... I really do believe condoms protect against it ... and the female condoms even more than the male condoms because they cover a larger surface area.

Maya also advocated for the inclusion of HPV sexual education programs as an integral component in secondary school curricula, but she felt that conversations about sex needed to happen on a societal level as well. Maya felt this should be the starting point, as many North Americans are uncomfortable talking about sex let alone contemplating sexual education programs in schools. This may, however, be in part because sexual education is rarely offered extensively in schools, she thought. As she discussed the circularity of this argument, she was quick to stress that she had not received any sexual education while in elementary or secondary school. Maya described her chats with fellow sexual health researchers in her graduate nursing program:

> I had very unsafe sexual practices when I was younger – very, very unsafe. And I guess I didn't really have any sexual health education, and it wasn't because my parents are right wing or anything like that. It was just kind of not talked about. Or maybe I didn't want to talk about it. I probably didn't at the time. I'm sure they tried and I told them to screw off or something like that.
>
> But then I had other friends that never had unsafe sex in their whole lives, which totally blows my mind. But then they had very proactive parents that from an early age were sort of ingraining this stuff into them, like, this is the science behind it. It's not scary, it's not a big deal – this is just what it means ... If I had maybe had more of the science ... I think it could have made me make different decisions, possibly.

In talking about increasing interpersonal and institutional conversations about sexual health education, Maya, like Sylvana, touched on the vulnerability of women while negotiating sexual encounters:

There's also the layer of young girls not being empowered to make these decisions as well. So, that has nothing to do with education. Like, you may know that having unsafe sex, unprotected sex, is dangerous, but that you don't necessarily have the power to make that choice in the situation. And so that adds another dimension to it.

This dimension, as Maya referred to it, was a theme that recurred throughout all of my interviews, regardless of whether or not the women were mothers negotiating the vaccine for their daughters or university students contemplating being vaccinated. The theme of vulnerability or lack of power while negotiating one's sexual health is explored in more detail in later on in this chapter.

Gender as It Bears upon HPV Vaccine Decision-Making

The lack of sexual education accompanying HPV vaccine policy in Ontario was not the only aspect of government programming that upset students; they were also, overwhelmingly, annoyed by the gendering of the vaccine. As Sylvana stated,

I think that what people should be emphasizing their preventative measures towards is a lot more screening and especially [for] males. There is a huge problem with males because apparently they, like in a lot of sexually transmitted diseases, do not show any symptoms whatsoever … and hav[e] no clue that they have an infection. So it is actually incorrect at this point to give vaccines to young children instead of funding research to screen people and then funding educational classes in schools.

Sylvana also pointed out that in addition to the lack of sexual health education available, men, in her experience, were tasked with the decision of whether or not to use a condom in a sexual relationship/encounter. This was a troubling trend for Sylvana that she would like to see changed; however, because altering such a complex sociocultural phenomenon would be a difficult task, it should be addressed in sexual health education.

Maya was more forceful in her discussion than Sylvana. She felt at a loss as to how to manage the complexity of issues surrounding the vaccine, particularly how to resolve the tension between the vulnerability of women negotiating their sexual health and the potential assistance that the vaccine could offer in spite of the outright targeting of women – targeting that becomes synonymous with blame when women acquire an STI. Maya elaborated on the dilemma caused by Gardasil advertising and provincial in-school vaccination programming:

Women are meant to feel, made to feel, bad about their bodies in so many different ways. And this is another way in which we're disempowering women to make healthy choices and to take their own health into their own hands by saying you need this vaccine because you're going to have sex, you're going to get dirty, it's going to make you sick. I think it can be done in a way that's empowering … but the way it's being marketed as a gendered vaccine is saying that the girls in our society are unhealthy, the girls in our society are intrinsically sexually deviant and are going to get STIs and the boys are not, and so here's some way to protect them, protect the virginity, protect the innocence of these girls from getting sullied with sexually trans-mitted diseases. And that just makes me sick thinking of it that way.

Maya was not the only one made to feel "sick" about the gendering of HPV. Amber, a twenty-six-year-old law student, was even more outraged than Sylvana and Maya. She is the first in her family to attend university and one of the few students I interviewed from a working-class back-ground. As our interview progressed, Amber became more and more agitated – in fact, her anger about these issues was clearly palpable by the end of our time together. Amber had a decided opinion with respect to the gendering of STIs:

I think it would be associated with the turn of the nineteenth century. To my knowledge a lot of issues about venereal disease had come up during this period and they were very much associated with women. Even though, as we know today, it takes two partners, it [STIs] is just still, I guess, associ-ated with female, dirty sexual behaviour.

Amber elaborated further:

When I was doing the research on the vaccine and HPV, one thing that they said was the reason why a lot of STDs [sexually transmitted diseases] and venereal diseases become associated with women is because oftentimes the symptoms appear on women as opposed to, and not so much, on men. And the reason for this being that the vagina is really hospitable for the growth of different bacteria and viruses.

Even though students exhibited consensus regarding their irritation with the gendering of the vaccine, this annoyance did not lead to uni-form decisions. Some students were so turned off by the gendering of the vaccine and what they perceived as potential vaccine risk in the absence of long-term data that they refused to get vaccinated. Others were mildly perturbed by the gendering and also worried about potential vaccine risks, but this only resulted in them putting off their decisions. Others grudgingly got vaccinated, but made it clear that this "choice" was by no means an endorsement of HPV vaccine gendering. Almost two thirds of the students interviewed decided not to be vaccinated or to delay vaccination decision-making. It should be noted that even though students were concerned about potential vaccine risk or long-term side effects, they were not anti-vaccine. Students, as was the case with the mothers, did not suggest that people should not get vaccinated at all, but rather that they should be cautious of new vaccines until longer-term research is released. Each of the three vaccine decisions is discussed in turn below.

Saying "No" to Gendering and Vaccine Risk

As concerned with sexual health as Maya was – this was after all the basis of her graduate training in nursing – she chose not to get vaccinated due to the gendering of the vaccine and what she perceived as vaccine risk. Maya explained her decision-making rationale:

> I'm really sceptical about the vaccine, particularly because it's mass marketed towards girls. I just feel that if we actually want to reduce cancer we probably should be vaccinating everyone … That they're targeting only girls and women [when] there hasn't been any long-term research on the effects of the vaccine … I think that's really problematic.
>
> I read recently that at least in the [United] States and some other countries the vaccine has now been approved for boys – I guess it hasn't been in Canada yet.[4] But there's no willingness or feeling like there's a need to promote it for boys and men the way that they have for girls and women. There's no mass campaign to get these boys vaccinated even though the vaccine is available, which I think is just crazy and just really telling.

In addition to being unsettled by the marketing of HPV as a women's disease, Maya was also concerned about long-term vaccine risks. She expanded further:

> Not to be like a conspiracy theorist … but what is being said is that it is okay to put women and girls at risk of a vaccine that we are not really sure what's going to happen in the long term or how effective it is actually in preventing cancer … but we're not going to take that risk with boys. I think that offering it for free is kind of pushing people in the direction of taking it, because you know if they don't get it that year then they are going to have to pay hundreds of dollars to get it. I think it's maybe a coerced choice, if it's a choice at all. This seems like not the best situation.

> I'm wary of anybody taking the vaccine. I'm under the impression that the vaccine was really expedited ... There are cases of medical intervention for women that have shown detrimental long-term health effects. You know, the birth control pill when it was first put out there had no long-term data, then we found out that people who take the pill for a long period of time have higher chances of stroke.

Saying "no" to the vaccine was Maya's way of saying "no" to the gendered risk discourses of the government and pharmaceutical companies. However, she was also saying "no" to women's over-medicalization. Not wanting to take the vaccine was an act taken to protect her health by avoiding, what was in her view, unnecessary risk. Instead, she managed the risk of further contracting STIs by using condoms and not engaging in unprotected sex unless both she and her partner had tested negative for STIs. Additionally, Maya attempted to stave off cervical cancer by getting regular Pap smears, which she arranged every year with her general practitioner (GP).

Morgan, an undergraduate liberal arts major, also declined vaccination. She did so for two reasons: what she viewed as the aggressive promotion of the vaccine by campus clinic physicians to female students and the potential risks associated with a relatively new vaccine. Morgan shares her experiences with Gardasil advertising and campus clinic physicians:

> We are pretty impressionable, so it's hard when you're getting a lot of people talking for it. Like, you see the ads and you talk to your doctors, at school especially, they're always prescribing it to you. I have told them that I do not want it. They're like, well, "I just couldn't live with myself if you came back here in six months' time with HPV because I didn't talk to you about the vaccine." I was like, "Okay, thanks," and I just threw it in my bag.

Morgan was further put off by the ubiquitous vaccine advertising on campus, which included a full-page advertisement in her university sponsored day planner and in campus washroom stalls, but she was also uncertain of the risks the vaccine could potentially bring. She elaborated:

> Most doctors do recommend it, but I just think that it doesn't really replace regular check-ups. I just think the implementation of it was really quick, so I am very wary of it. I don't think that five, seven years is a long enough trial if you don't know any of the long-term effects now.

The pressure that Morgan felt to get vaccinated from multiple sources as well as concerns for the potential risk a relatively new vaccine could bring were also keenly felt by those who delayed vaccination.

Delaying Decision-Making Due to Vaccine Risk

While Sylvana was still recovering from the shock of discovering she had genital warts, she was contemplating getting the HPV vaccine. She was not sure whether she would reach a decision any time soon. As she frequently mentioned, she had "really mixed thoughts" about the vaccine, and she talked about the problems the vaccine presented for her:

> It's very difficult to navigate this debate as a woman who is concerned about these things [her health] personally … You're trying to balance all the social factors – the government, pharmaceutical, physiological … they're really complicated. I think part of my problem [re: decision-making] is that I am so lost in this analysis.

Sylvana balanced worries about her own health with her desire not to acquiesce to vaccine marketing and policy that targeted women without considering HPV within the context of gender relations. There was a tug of war between her individual concerns and the "bigger picture." Sylvana saw this picture as one that painted women in a subordinate, needy, and risky position vis-à-vis HPV, and this was reflective of her general social position – a position subordinate to men. As Sylvana said, "it's just women who have to make sure that you prevent yourself from getting into trouble, or you have to make sure you're taking the pill and that kind of thing to make sure you are not getting pregnant. It's always the woman who has to do those." Sylvana was pointing out that women must take social responsibility for their bodies and yet are blamed for not protecting themselves.

Sylvana delayed decision-making primarily because of the gendering of the vaccine, but her perspective was further complicated by her distrust of pharmaceutical companies:

> They say they [Gardasil] have been proven to reduce the risks of HPV. But … there are so many types of HPV. So, what is it – [strains] 6, 11, 16, and 18 that it protects? Now, 4 out of 100, that's 4 per cent – that's huge to even just say that it protects you from HPV. Maybe those are the more prominent ones – you know what I mean, there's not too much information about that, right? Maybe those are the ones that are easier to fight off. Maybe we might get them one day from having sexual intercourse and you just fight them off. But it's not talked about, right? My boss's niece got the vaccine and she still got warts. That's why I don't really trust vaccines. What it essentially is, I get it, is a cash grab by a pharma company. They're in the business of selling you stuff that you don't necessarily need.

Not only was Sylvana sceptical of the necessity of the HPV vaccine, but she was also wary of its benefits, considering that it covers only 4 out of 100 HPV strains. For Sylvana, claims that the HPV vaccine protects women from cancer were an overblown marketing strategy.

Lison, an undergraduate liberal arts major, also delayed making her HPV vaccine decision. Like Madeleine, Lison has experienced cervical dysplasia and must return to her physician every six months for Pap testing in order to monitor the trajectory of her abnormal cervical cells. This has been going on for a few years now. Negative media coverage surrounding the vaccine was part of Lison's decision to delay the vaccine. She explains:

> I don't know if it was here or in the United States … but a lot of girls were getting sick from it or just having really bad side effects … It just worries me, that stuff – I don't know if it is true what the media [says] or what was in the news about girls getting sick from it. I don't know if someone died from it or if they made that up, I don't know. I would have to learn more about it before I would make a clear decision where I am going to fall.

It is important to stress that students who delayed making a decision were deeply conflicted about the vaccine. Balancing individual health needs with their distaste for the overarching negative messaging in pharmaceutical advertising and Ontario government policy was a difficult task indeed. They were also hyperaware of the negative media coverage surrounding HPV vaccine risk and found it difficult to ascertain which news stories were factual. As Sylvana said, "It's a hard kind of choice to make. But at the same time, how stupid would you feel if you ended up getting cervical cancer and had decided not to get vaccinated."

Saying "Yes" to the Vaccine

While the students who decided to get vaccinated were in the minority, they all shared common motivations. Experiencing HPV infection, or knowing someone who had, was the most common impetus. Madeleine had had three STIs and undergone a LEEP. While uncertain if the vaccine would be of benefit to her, she did support vaccinating girls before they become sexually active, with the proviso that HPV informational programming accompany the shot. Madeleine felt it was important to emphasize that the vaccine does not protect against all HPV strains and that it isn't a "full-plan condom."

As my interview with Amber was winding down, I was surprised to learn that she did indeed get vaccinated against HPV. Amber's decision was a bit startling considering how passionately she spoke out against the gendering of STIs, HPV, and the vaccine, but also because she had condemned the vaccine a year earlier in a blog entry (which she brought along to our interview). The blog post reads:

> To all my women readers out there: don't get the HPV vaccine! Seriously, this is just a grab by big pharma to target and stigmatize women for a virus that has little chance of actually turning into cancer. That's right – HPV does not necessarily turn into cancer. Don't buy into the hype. Our bodies don't need to represent disease. We are not the bearers of ill health and "dirty" viruses. Resist this continual characterization of women by saying "no." Say "no" to this egregious portrayal of women and big pharma profits.[5]

Amber's blog entry and her decision to be vaccinated seem incongruous. However, the inconsistency points to the complexity of vaccine decision-making for women. Amber's decision is not necessarily a reversal of her position on the gendering of STIs, HPV, and the vaccine but instead reflects the theme of sexual health vulnerability, as discussed by Sylvana and Maya earlier in this chapter. Amber explained:

> I have a problem ... with the vaccine even though I got it ... because the way it's being marketed towards girls stigmatizes girls' and women's sexualities ... it puts the onus on girls. Just like when you look at having responsible, protective sex, again a lot of the onus is put on girls to be sort of the arbitrators of sexuality, so that they have to monitor their partner's behaviour and make sure to take on that responsibility ... for both her and her partner without attributing very much responsibility to the man who is involved in the sexual relationship.

Despite Amber's strong reservations about the social consequences of vaccine marketing and policy, it was personal experience that brought about her change in decision-making. Learning that a friend had contracted an HPV infection, Amber conducted some research:

> One thing that I found was it's very difficult to prevent the contraction of HPV when your partner has it ... even with the use of condoms. And I guess that's probably because the virus itself doesn't exist explicitly on the reproductive organs.[6]
>
> Having seen my friend going through having HPV, I think it's a pretty terrible thing to go through ... it's going to affect how her relationships end up unravelling and that sort of thing and whom she meets. I guess my own concern about my sexual health outweighed any of the potential problems that might come with it.

Students like Amber are actively conscious of the societal challenges the current, gendered HPV vaccine policy and marketing in Canada bring, but ultimately their own sense of sexual health vulnerability takes precedence over these misgivings. The complexity of vaccine decision-making was made abundantly clear to me after witnessing Amber's conflict over her decision to get vaccinated. The influence of adverse HPV experiences relayed by friends, family, and colleagues served as a strong motivator for women to get the vaccination.

De-gendering and De-individualization

Students were developing their sense of self, their ethical identities, by doing gender through resistance to being put in a box of the "feminine" (Moore 2010, 96) by sales/governance strategies. The students I interviewed were upset and angry with the gendering of the vaccine and the virus to the extent that 70 per cent decided against vaccination or delayed their decision.[7] The decision to forgo vaccination is a form of what Pieter Streefland, A.M.R. Chowdry, and Pilar Ramos-Jimenez (1999, 1710) call "non-acceptance," where individuals "question the need for vaccination." When non-acceptance becomes widespread, collective resistance can emerge, such as the nineteenth-century grassroots campaign against smallpox vaccination in England. But for these students, decision-making occurred on an individual level where there was "no organization, no active mobilization" (Streefland, Chowdry, and Ramos-Jimenez 1999, 1712).

Interestingly, though, in explaining their reasoning for non-acceptance, students moved from the individualized sphere of vaccine decision-making to seeking collective measures to address vaccine gendering and its social consequences. As Maya stated, the gendering of the vaccine and STIs made her feel "sick." Sylvana described this type of gendering as "the wrong approach." Amber felt that contemporary gendering was a continuation of negative historical discourses vis-à-vis women that could be traced back to the nineteenth century. Maya's decision not to get the vaccine and Sylvana's decision to delay were both ways of saying "no" to the gendering of the vaccine (and the virus) in governmental and pharmaceutical discourses.[8] Even Amber, who changed her mind in favour of being vaccinated after seeing a friend experience a protracted HPV infection, was conscious of the social implications that gendered HPV vaccine policy and pharmaceutical sales/governance strategies brought. As Jessica Gregg (2011, 77) notes, "STDs are ... particularly stigmatizing for women, for whom cultural ideals of premarital virginity, marital monogamy, and respectability clash with the reality of sexually transmitted infections."

Sylvana and Maya resisted the subject formation of the risky HPV-related girl/woman by saying "no" to the vaccine, but at the same time they were acutely aware of gender imbalances in sexual health negotiation. As such, their vaccine negotiation was rife with "paradox" (Butler 2004, 3) and complexity similar to that which mothers experienced. Students spoke in great detail about the challenge of negotiating sexual health (see Richens, Imrie, and Weiss 2003; Roche, Neaigus, and Miller 2005; Shoveller et al. 2010; Thomas 2005) where gender imbalances brought risk into their daily lives. In practice, as Sylvana explained, women experience vulnerability, even where they believe themselves to be in a monogamous sexual relationship. While open communication between partners is ideal, Sylvana experienced a breakdown in such communication when her partner was unfaithful and she was left, as she said, "exposed."

Maya also spoke about the vulnerability young women experience in sexual encounters:

> But then there's also the layer of young girls not being empowered to make these decisions as well. So, that has nothing to do with education. Like you may know that having unsafe sex, unprotected sex, is dangerous, but you don't necessarily have the power to make that choice in the situation.

Like Maya, students did not always feel they had the power to press for the use of barrier contraceptives while engaging in sexual practices without alienating a male partner. This, coupled with the fact that partners were not always faithful, made students feel vulnerable. While Maya's and Sylvana's decision not to be vaccinated can be placed within the frame of doing gender through resistance, Amber's "yes" can also be viewed as a form of quiet protest. Amber deployed vaccination as a tool to help strengthen her position in future sexual health negotiation. Amber revealed, "My own concern about my sexual health outweighed any potential problems that might come with it." Students thus demonstrated that resistance was as intricate as the paradoxes exhibited by mothers and that it could not be measured by vaccine decision outcomes alone.

Overall, students urged for a more open climate about sex, sexual relations, and STIs. They reasoned that if more people talked openly about sex, sexual health negotiation would be more balanced, with both men and women taking measures to protect themselves. Offering the HPV vaccine in school settings without providing accompanying sexual health education struck them as a missed opportunity. They were convinced that if sexual education was covered more frequently and in more depth in both primary and secondary schools, not only would young women be aided in negotiating their sexual health, but it would also help lift the STI-related "stigma" (Goffman 1963). As more individuals realize how commonplace STIs are, the compulsion to remain silent for fear of being judged could lift.

By wanting to bring sex and sexual relations into everyday conversation, students were not only aiming to ease the stigma – they were trying to resist it. This was an effort in reordering daily discourse. Through reordering, they resisted the social exclusion that resulted from others knowing they had contracted an STI and being depicted as "dirty" or "deviant" women. As Veena Das (2001) writes, in terms of disability,

> the stigma of deformed bodies … is about reduction of sociality, exclusion from moral community as well as subjective feelings of guilt and shame. Being cast out of the social community coupled with a diminished sense of worth reduces the capability of the afflicted person to seek help. (5)

Student resistance to the gendering of the vaccine and the virus, their vulnerability in sexual health negotiation, and the stigma associated with STIs were all factors integral to their developing sense of self as young women. Their telos involved rejecting being painted as "dirty" and "sexualized," even while being acutely concerned about the uneven power relations present in sexual health negotiation with male partners. This was a complex form of risk negotiation involving refusing outright to be identified as risky sexual beings while trying to find ways to mitigate risk as sexually active women who had contracted STIs.

Their prescription for dealing with stigma was increased sexual health education, both in schools and in society in general through public health measures. Students attempted to adjust the neo-liberal devolution of public health services, which has been rampant under the auspices of the new public health paradigm (Lupton and Petersen 1996), by urging for greater sexual health education in schools. As such, students were trying to shift the onus for public health education from the individual back onto the state.[9] Their negotiation of risk thus involved a reordering of existing power structures. As with mothers, there was "no self-making outside of the norms that orchestrate the possible forms that a subject may take" (Butler 2008, 26–7). This speaks to the recognition that risk is a social product: if it can be constructed as an individual and gendered problem through sales/governance strategies, these premises can also be deconstructed through state provided educational programming.

Managing Risk, Uncertainty, and Trust in Vaccine Decision-Making

Students were also doing a form of risk through living with intermittent HPV infections. Their risk came and went partly because of the strength of the immune system at their relatively young ages, which can typically clear HPV infections that cause cervical dysplasia on its own. Moreover, medical treatments for genital warts ensured that these types of infections did not last long, and genital warts are the result of low-risk HPV strains, which do not lead to cancer.

These intermittent experiences caused students to enact their own forms of telos in order to mitigate future HPV infection risk. For example, Maya managed her sexual health by engaging in sex only with barrier protection unless she and her partner had received negative STI tests. She used condoms when necessary and had a Pap test at her yearly physical with her GP. These active strategies helped Maya manage sexual health negotiation and keep an eye out for dysplasia. Maya refused the HPV vaccine because of its associated gendering and the potential risks of a new vaccine. As she stated, "I don't know how anybody can expose themselves to a drug that they don't know how it's going to affect them in the long term. I think that's kind of crazy, so I wouldn't advocate for anybody taking the vaccine."

The absence of long-term studies leads to the "question of *deciding in a context of uncertainty*" (Giddens 1991, 217; emphasis in original). In a time of uncertainty, trust is at issue. According to Giddens (1991, 18), in order to trust in late modernity, particularly in the case of new technical and medical developments, an individual must have a sense of psychological "security." Continually emerging risks work to destabilize this. The "protective cocoon" that is required in order to go out into the world on a daily basis and partake in everyday risk inducing activities, such as driving a car or crossing the street, can be harder and harder to maintain in times of uncertainty (40). The "bracketing-out of possible events or issues which could, in certain circumstances, be cause for alarm" is no longer necessarily possible (127). In short, if an individual's sense of "basic trust is fragile ... even contemplating a small risk, particularly in relation to a highly cherished aim, may prove intolerable" (182).

The notion of trust took on various gradations in relation to vaccine decision-making for students. Sylvana, for example, had difficulty trusting pharmaceutical companies. She was wary of, as she said, "putting stuff in my body that I don't know exactly what it is and what is does ... What it essentially is, I get it, is a cash grab by a pharma company." It is not uncommon for individuals to mistrust medical products that have been developed by for-profit entities, because positive notions of health and health care are more often associated with non-profit spheres (Gross and Shuval 2008, 553). However, to feel at risk after having experienced multiple HPV infections, and then having been made to feel further at risk by a medical solution, such as the vaccine, left Sylvana at a loss. This translated into a delayed decision regarding the vaccine. Amber, on the other hand, demonstrated enough trust to undergo vaccination, even though she did not agree with the sales/governance strategies used to promote it. Student experiences demonstrate that trust is a nuanced and layered concept. And, as is exemplified by Amber's change of heart (her initial decision to forgo vaccination was reversed when a close friend experienced HPV-related complications), trust can also be dynamic and changing. As Walls et al. (2010, 147) explain, "critical trust lies on a continuum between outright skepticism (rejection) and uncritical emotional acceptance."

Conclusion

The pain, shame, and anxiety attached to having an STI, and the few appropriate social channels through which to express these feelings and experiences, had clearly taken a toll on the young women interviewed. Students wanted to reframe how STIs were viewed in society. Instead of being considered a traumatic experience event, students wished that HPV infection could be positioned as part and parcel of a regular sexually active life. As HPV infection cannot be prevented, most sexually active individuals will contract a strain of the virus during their lifetime, as had Sylvana, Maya, Madeleine, and Lison. Thus, they argued, it is unnecessary to level stigma. However, at the same time, students such as Sylvana felt that they were vulnerable to catching STIs from unfaithful partners. After she discovered her boyfriend had cheated on her, Sylvana delayed making a decision about the HPV vaccine in order to first determine if he would be faithful to her in the future. As such, students were concerned about not being able to successfully negotiate their own sexual health in their heterosexual relationships.

Overall, students called for more open communication surrounding sexual activity, whether it was as part of a couple, between peers, or within popular discourses. Maya and Madeleine advocated for sexual education to be an integral component of secondary school curriculum, particularly when the HPV vaccine is offered in schools. Students wanted to increase interpersonal and institutional conversations about sex.

The majority of students chose not to be vaccinated or delayed making their decision. Their outrage at the gendering of the vaccine directly influenced their vaccine decision-making to some extent. Those who chose not to be vaccinated were also concerned about potential long-term vaccine side effects. As the vaccine was relatively new, no long-term studies regarding the vaccine were available, and the potentiality of the vaccine itself to bring forth risk was too big a chance to take. Those who chose to be vaccinated did so because they or someone they knew had contracted cervical dysplasia, which required medical intervention. These inoculated students wanted to avoid undergoing the same stressful and devastating experiences that friends and relatives had undergone. However, the decision to be vaccinated did not diminish concerns about the social impact of the gendering of the vaccine. Amber was acutely aware of increased stigma being levelled against women who were infected with HPV without the same critique being directed at men, but she deemed that mitigating her sexual health vulnerability through vaccination was a higher priority.

In sum, while navigating HPV vaccine decision-making, students were actively fashioning their ethical beings or senses of self. As women emerging into full-fledged womanhood, students were attempting to mediate gendered stereotypes associated with STIs by advocating for the de-gendering of the vaccine. They were also strongly critiquing neoliberal public health measures, which place the onus for sexual health education and negotiation on the individual. These themes were central to how they each identified as a woman – they wanted to be considered on equal footing with men and thus declined a vaccine they associated with gender asymmetry. While it was clear what type of women they wished to be, actually mediating HPV infection risk and the potential risks of the vaccine proved to be rife with uncertainty. Students had begun to experience intermittent HPV infections but felt that the vaccine was too "new" to be trusted. Opposition to big pharma and uncertainty surrounding vaccine side effects caused students anxiety. They felt vulnerable to vaccine risks – just as exposed as they felt while negotiating their own sexual health. Thus, for students, the concept of situated risk was fraught with continual negotiation. Being a strong, certain woman in the face of mistrust and uncertainty was a difficult and tenuous ideal to actualize.

4 Media Landscape: Controversies and Competing Narratives

Introduction

All of the women I interviewed were confronted with having to make a challenging personal decision against a backdrop of competing messaging and considerable public resistance. While Merck Frosst was successful in its influence over HPV vaccine policymaking, negative public commentary and media coverage of the vaccine roll-out was immediate and swift. Much of the negative coverage stemmed from an August 2007 *Maclean's* cover story titled, "Our Girls Are Not Guinea Pigs" (Gulli 2007). Public debate took a "What's the hurry?" (Mah et al. 2011) approach centred on the notion that while the vaccine might prove effective in curbing cervical cancer, this could not be determined until long-term data emerged. Public health worked hard at redirecting this narrative to little success. The Public Health Agency of Canada (PHAC) released statements stressing the agency backed the vaccine as an effort in preventative care. Public health officials also released HPV vaccine research and were active in pushing back in the media. These strategies came to a crux in the winter of 2015 with a *Toronto Star* exposé questioning the safety of the vaccine. Public health officials across Canada responded with a letter condemning this media coverage, which resulted in the *Toronto Star* apologizing and removing the original story from the public record. Despite all these public health communication efforts, HPV vaccine uptake is still below targets in Ontario today.

To gather the data for this chapter, I inputted the search term "HPV vaccine" into the media database Factiva. The search time frame was from 1 January 2007 to 30 June 2016, which resulted in 1,471 entries. Duplicate articles were removed as were press releases, including corporate communications issued directly by pharmaceutical companies and related lobby groups, resulting in a total of 491 news articles deemed

Table 1. Canadian HPV vaccine media coverage and story trends, 2007–16

Year	Total Articles	Positive	Negative	Neutral
2007	153	73	28	52
2008	103	47	29	27
2009	39	22	9	8
2010	11	10	0	1
2011	22	20	1	1
2012	34	24	6	4
2013	26	25	1	0
2014	25	22	1	2
2015	59	54	5	0
2016	19	18	1	0

relevant for analysis (see Table 1). The volume of non-news items collected by Factiva's search result is significant at 33 per cent. This points to the active communications deployed on behalf of pharmaceutical manufacturers and related organizations. Lobbying efforts were also apparent where heads of physician groups who received grant money from Merck Frosst were prominently displayed and quoted in news coverage. The news items, both articles and TV transcripts, were analysed using a critical discourse analysis approach (Henry and Tator 2002, 71–7; Leiss, Kline, and Jhally 1990, 197–224) in order to determine which issues were being reported upon and how these "stories" were framed (Cairney 2012, 175).

Mass media is but one site of discourse that creates and perpetuates the "risky girl/woman" stereotype and works to perpetuate this "truth." As per Foucault (1994, 31), truths operate in a triangular constellation of "power, right, truth," which results in the circulation of discursive "facts" that reinforce the right to govern in a certain manner, thereby reinforcing the status quo. Analogously, Pierre Bourdieu (1977, 164) argues that "systems of classification which produce ... classes, i.e. divisions by sex, age, or position ... make their specific contribution to the reproduction of power relations of which they are the product." For Bourdieu, "the theory of knowledge is a dimension of political theory because of the specifically symbolic power to impose the principles of the construction of reality – in particular, social reality – is a major dimension of political power" (164). As such, the analysis below reinforces how power is instituted through binaries in the propagation of truths. These binaries are built upon false dichotomies of the at-risk female vs. the healthy male, good citizens who vaccinate vs. bad citizens who do not, fiction vs. science, and anti-vaccine vs. pro-vaccine, all of

which littered news coverage of the HPV vaccine in Canada for close
to a decade. In short, media coverage of the vaccine is divisive, with
several story arcs illustrating how hard public health officials worked
to control a narrative that very much ran the risk of veering off its intended course.

Gendered Endorsement Leitmotif and the "What's the Hurry?" Response (2007)

In 2007, with the vaccine's roll-out across the country, media coverage
was voluminous. Of the 153 articles surveyed, 47.7 per cent portrayed
positive views of the vaccine, 18 per cent projected "negative" views,
and 33.9 per cent adopted a neutral tone. Among the articles deemed
positive were two common narrative strategies: the first highlighted the
endorsement of the vaccine by numerous Canadian governmental agencies, Canadian medical societies, and individual physicians; the second
showcased the potential risk of HPV through the narratives of women in
their twenties diagnosed with cervical cancer. Significantly, only a small
smattering of stories in 2007 addressed the gendering of the vaccine by
asking why it was not offered to boys.

The endorsement narrative strategy was featured in 25 per cent of
articles tagged as positive. The endorsements referenced largely recy-
cled medical society press releases or position papers recommending
the vaccine to school-age girls. For example, the Canadian Paediatric
Society's endorsement was immediately apparent in an *Ottawa Citizen*
headline, which read, "Pediatricians Group Backs HPV Vaccine for
Girls; Recommends Shot for Nine- to 13-Year-Olds" (Kubacki 2007).
Modified versions of the same story by Maria Kubacki were syndicated
in Canwest papers across the country. The article began by referring to
the Canadian Paediatric Society as a "group representing more than
2,500 pediatricians across Canada," giving the impression that an overwhelming number of paediatricians supported the vaccination of girls.
Earlier in the year, on 19 March, the Canadian Pharmacists Association lauded the federal government for their financial support in fa-
cilitating the delivery of the vaccine by the provinces (Canadian Press
2007a). This article included contact details for the public affairs man-
ager of the Association. On 21 June, the *Vancouver Sun* reported that
the Society of Obstetricians and Gynaecologists of Canada (SOGC) recommended the vaccine (Laucius 2007a), and in response to "negative"
media coverage the vaccine received in 2007, a commentary piece appeared in the *Globe and Mail* on 11 September in which representatives
of the Society of Gynecologic Oncoloy of Canada (GOC) expressed

concern "that the recent rhetoric surrounding the human papilloma-virus (HPV) vaccine has the potential to derail a major advance in pre-vention of cervical cancer and its precursors" (Fung-Kee-Fung et al. 2007).

Several articles that appeared in 2007 highlighted governmental or-ganizations or high-ranking employees who urged vaccine uptake. The *National Post* ran a story on 31 January highlighting the National Advi-sory Committee on Immunization's (NACI) recommendation that girls aged nine to thirteen be vaccinated (Kirkey 2007). The article began with the lead, "Every nine- to 13-year-old girl in the country should be vaccinated against the sexually transmitted virus that causes cervical can-cer," and went on to say that "studies suggest 10% to 29% of women in Canada are infected with HPV, making it the most common sexually transmitted infection in the country. Infants can also be exposed to the virus from their mother's genital tract." These messages were echoed in an article in the *Waterloo Region Record* that same day, as well as a day later in an article in the *Hamilton Spectator* (2007), both "urging" that girls nine to thirteen get the vaccine. Endorsements also followed from lo-cal medical officers of health in Vancouver and Ottawa (Canadian Press 2007b; Parks and Salisbury 2007), as well as from Cancer Care Ontario's director of screening (Mai 2007). While these endorsements were to be expected, it is notable that both the *Montreal Gazette* (2007) and the *Globe and Mail* (2007) endorsed the vaccine in their op-ed and editorial columns.

In provoking a fear of cancer in its readers, media sources further en-dorsed the vaccine. The risk of cervical cancer was often presented with-out the necessary context by which to gage one's potential likelihood of acquiring it. For example, an article in the *Guelph Mercury* (2007) on 20 October stated that the "Canadian Cancer Society estimates 1,350 Cana-dian women will get cervical cancer this year and 390 will die from the disease. While the numbers may seem small, Aoki [a University of Mani-toba researcher] was quoted ... as saying some women who contract cer-vical cancer from HPV cannot be treated with chemotherapy, radiation, or surgery." Other stories included testimonies of women diagnosed with cervical cancer. In a *National Post* piece that appeared on 24 Sep-tember, Ms. Lewis, a forty-six-year-old cervical cancer survivor who had undergone surgery, radiation, and chemotherapy, was quoted as saying, "For the people who say, 'Well, it's not deadly enough, the numbers are not there for the attention and money being poured into the vaccine,' I would say 'Wait until your sister or your daughter or your wife does get cervical cancer, then start talking about the numbers'" (Blackwell 2007). In the same article, Liz Elwood, a twenty-five-year-old who had recently been diagnosed with cervical cancer, stated, "It breaks my heart that girls could be getting this virus still, with some of them ultimately getting cancer, and we could be stopping it" (Blackwell 2007).

Interestingly, only three of the "positive" stories for 2007 discussed gender and the vaccine. Stories from the *Edmonton Journal* (Roan 2007), the *Globe and Mail* (Picard 2007), and the *Calgary Herald* (Keenan 2007) highlighted that boys and men do contract HPV and could benefit from vaccination. The *Calgary Herald* piece questioned the PHAC's position, stating it had failed to include research conducted in the United States, including two studies by Merck Frosst suggesting that the vaccine is effective in "stimulating antibodies" in males (Keenan 2007). Merck Frosst and government policy branded HPV a women's issue, as discussed in chapters 5 and 6. This chapter demonstrates that the national media did so as well.

The endorsement articles, as well as those that framed the vaccine as a cancer fighter by highlighting individual stories, were countered with what public health officials would deem "negative" media coverage, which was blamed for low uptake rates in Ontario when the vaccine was introduced in 2007. However, upon close examination, these articles advocated a "What's the hurry?" (Mah et al. 2011) approach. A significant portion of coverage in 2007 – 18 per cent of the articles surveyed – brought forth questions about the vaccine and the need to introduce a mass vaccination program so quickly. Of this "negative" coverage, 92 per cent advocated for more research into the vaccine's efficacy and safety before programs were rolled out. A representative example of the bulk of the "negative" coverage can be seen in a letter to the editor of the *Ottawa Citizen* on 21 March by McGill University professor Dr. Abby Lippman, then chair of the Canadian Women's Health Network (CWHN). Lippman (2007) wrote, "Until we know lots more about the vaccine, as well as how effective it actually is in reducing cervical cancer rates, health-care dollars may be better spent in enhancing pap screening programs (including pap registries), and ensuring they reach the most marginalized populations."

Lippman's work on the HPV vaccine, including papers for the CWHN (2007) and the *Canadian Medical Association Journal* (Lippman et al. 2007), was often cited in media stories questioning the speedy roll-out of the school-based vaccination programming. A story appearing in the *Calgary Herald* on 2 August quoted Lippman as saying, "Take a deep breath. We don't have a crisis or an epidemic" (Laucius 2007b). Margaret Wente (2007) took a similar approach in her column in the *Globe and Mail* on 14 August, stating, "Cervical cancer isn't exactly polio. It is in no way an epidemic. It is a rare cancer that, thanks to Pap smears, is already well controlled. It accounts for less than 1 per cent of all cancer deaths. Lung cancer kills 25 times more women every year." While Lippman's arguments were taken up by journalists, her commentary in the *Canadian Medical Association Journal* (*CMAJ*) was critiqued by physicians in a multi-authored response published in a subsequent issue (Franco et al. 2007). The SOGC also went on record to say they were "disappointed" with Lippman's piece in *CMAJ*, stating that the "arguments expressed in this commentary lack grounding in scientific evidence" (Talaga 2007).

The "What's the hurry?" coverage also pointed out that the swift introduction of the vaccine was due to strong lobbying efforts on the part of the manufacturer, Merck Frosst. As Shelley Page (2007b) wrote in a piece for the *Vancouver Sun* on 14 May:

> The process has been so tainted by one drug company pursuing its own commercial interests that it's difficult to know whether financing the HPV vaccine is the right decision from a public health perspective. It might well be, but the heavy lobbying effort, from a former aide to Prime Minister Stephen Harper on down, muddles the debate.

The former aide Page was referring to is Ken Boessenkool, whom Tanya Talaga (2007) likewise named in her *Toronto Star* article on Merck Frosst's HPV vaccine lobbying efforts on 16 August. But Talaga went a step further, identifying other Hill+Knowlton staff who were working on the file, including Bob Lopinski, a former aide to Ontario Premier Dalton McGuinty, and Jason Grier, a former chief of staff to then Ontario Health Minister George Smitherman. "The speed with which ... Gardasil got onto both the federal and provincial political agendas was no accident," Talaga wrote.

One article published in August of 2007 remains controversial to this day. The *Maclean's* cover story "Our Girls Are Not Guinea Pigs" (Gulli 2007) set off a flurry of media coverage. The August print edition featured a shot of a single white "tween" girl with light brown hair, many freckles, and ruddy cheeks. She has a serious and almost defiant look on her face, which takes up most of the cover with only a bit of accompanying text. This lack of text renders the photo of the girl the most prominent feature on the cover. The article begins with a gripping anecdote of a girl who experienced side effects – headache, neck and back pain, and fever – attributed to the vaccine. The article's author, Cathy Gulli, adopts Lippman's concern about rolling out the vaccination program too soon:

Nearly every province in Canada has, in recent weeks, put forth some plan to implement an HPV vaccination program that will see the mass inoculation of an entire generation of girls ... with no serious acknowledgment of the potential health risks they may face. While everyone debates the moral and political consequences of endorsing Gardasil, the fundamental, essential medical and scientific debate remains untouched. So, in a few weeks, when thousands of girls concerned about Facebook and who will be in their class this year – not HPV – go back to school, many will become part of the biggest Canadian science experiment in decades. They will be guinea pigs. (Gulli 2007)

While Gulli was, no doubt, well-meaning, her portrayal of young female bodies as vulnerable, innocent, and asexual is problematic. Gulli could have easily questioned the science behind the vaccine and the data gaps mentioned by Lippman without invoking such gendered stereotypes. This story elicited a swift response from the PHAC. On 17 September, Dr. Butler-Jones (2007), then head of the PHAC, wrote a letter to the editor of the *Globe and Mail* titled, "What Happened to 'An Ounce of Prevention?'" He pointed out that, as a society, we tend to debate preventative measures, such as adding fluoride to drinking water and introducing vaccines, rather than treatment protocols. He argued that it is the role of public health to "improve the health of Canadians, to protect them and to reduce inequalities – including providing access to care, treatment and prevention." He also added a financial rationale, emphasizing that the prevention of disease is an "effective complement to an overburdened health-care system." This letter became news itself when medical reporter Helen Branswell (2007) of the Canadian Press interviewed Butler-Jones and quoted him as saying, "To suggest that this is some grand experiment is inappropriate ... There is no way we would do that sort of thing. You don't do that. It's totally unethical."

Before turning to the media coverage for 2008, it is worth noting that a third of the media coverage (34 per cent) in 2007 was deemed "neutral." By neutral, I am referring to balanced coverage that lists the pros and cons of the vaccine as they were understood in 2007 and offers context through which women can make informed decisions. The complex and varied mediascape (Appadurai 1990) – from those strongly advocating for the vaccine through medical endorsements and stories of those affected by cervical cancer to those arguing that inoculation campaigns were rushed, without sufficient research into vaccine safety and efficacy, and pushed by the profit motive of big pharma – is certainly a challenging information backdrop from which to draw and make health decisions.

Negative Coverage Focusing on Potential Vaccine Risks Gains Traction (2008)

Media coverage of the vaccine was still substantial in 2008 but had begun to wane. Of the 103 suitable media pieces that were analysed for 2008, 45 per cent were positive, 28 per cent were negative, and 26 per cent were classified as providing neutral coverage. Negative coverage of the vaccine had thus increased 10 per cent from 2007 to 2008, while positive and neutral coverage had both decreased. Much of the negative coverage had shifted to focus on potential side effects, which foreshadows the interviews with mothers and university-aged women students seen in chapters 2 and 3. For example, the *Victoria Times Colonist* (2008) reported on 2 September that the vaccine could potentially cause allergic reactions. The article opens by stating that "new safety data is linking the cervical cancer vaccine with a significantly higher than expected rate of anaphylaxis, a severe allergic reaction that can be life-threatening." An article published on the same day in the *Globe and Mail*, entitled "Allergy to HPV Vaccine Is Rare, but Still Dangerous, Australian Study Finds," uses an academic study to bolster the story angle. Referring to the vaccine as "controversial," the article's author, Tu Thanh Ha (2008), cites an Australian study, which had concluded that while the vaccine "triggers more severe allergic reactions than other vaccines ... the risk is still so tiny that HPV inoculation remains worthwhile." Ha goes on to write, however, that "the research was done on a small number of incidents, limiting its statistical clout." The article focuses on the case of a young Australian woman who contracted pancreatitis a few days after her first dose of the vaccine. The linkage is uncertain, but Ha nonetheless states that "despite the cautious tone of the Australian researchers, their findings may add fuel to the debate in Canada over HPV immunization."

An additional batch of negative articles considering potential risks of the vaccine were anchored around the opposition of the Catholic Bishops in Alberta, who argued that it was too soon to be vaccinating young girls given that the safety and efficacy of the vaccine had yet to be established. In a piece entitled "Does Vaccine Turn Girls into Guinea Pigs?" that ran on 28 October in the *Calgary Herald*, Bishop Fred Henry (2008) questioned the vaccine's safety. He quoted Dr. Diane M. Harper, physician, professor, and former director of the Gynaecological Cancer Prevention Research Group at Dartmouth Medical School: "This vaccine should not be mandated for 11-year-old girls ... it's not been tested in little girls for efficacy. At 11, these girls don't get cervical cancer – they won't know for 25 years if they will get cervical cancer. Giving it to 11-year-olds is a great big public health experiment." The bishop then refers to the 2007 *Maclean's* cover story that suggested adoption of the Gardasil vaccine would make "guinea pigs" of Canadian girls. It should be noted that Dr. Harper later received negative press for speaking out against the vaccine in the United States, including in response to a 2013 appearance on the *Katie Couric Show*. Katie Couric subsequently apologized that the episode failed to offer balanced reporting on the vaccine (Jaslow 2013).

There was some media mention on the vaccine in relation to men, including a *National Post* story on 14 November entitled "HPV Vaccine Prevents Genital Lesions in Men, Merck Study Claims." The article notes that the study "was funded by Merck, Gardasil's manufacturer," and Dr. Cassells, a University of Victoria researcher, is quoted as stating, "In order to sell the vaccine, you've got to sell the size of the problem" (Cowan 2008).

A significant portion of the positive coverage in 2008 focused on expanding subsidized vaccine coverage to young women and men beyond existing school-based programs. The *National Post*, for example, featured an article entitled "Vaccine Could End Most Cervical Cancer: Study; HPV Shots Urged for Older Women." This refers to a University of Ottawa study that urged the government to fund the vaccine for females ages fourteen to twenty-six. One of the study authors stated that "eradication could come quite easily ... All you really have to do is release a little bit of the vaccine into the adult population and you'd have it" (quoted in Blackwell 2008). An article published seven months later in the *Globe and Mail* carried the headline, "Merck-Sponsored Study Suggests HPV Vaccine Benefits Men Too." One of the study authors, Dr. Giuliano, is quoted as saying, "Gardasil prevents infection and disease at a very high level in males – that's the other half of the world" (quoted in M. Fox 2008). The article mentions that Merck Frosst was preparing to seek regulatory approval for the use of Gardasil in males based on research that indicated it reduced the incidence of genital warts and pre-cancerous penile lesions. An additional Associated Press (2008) file story released that same day also highlighted research indicating that the vaccine prevented genital warts in males, noting that "results are expected to bolster a likely bid by the vaccine manufacturer, Merck & Co. Inc., to begin marketing the vaccine to boys."

Not all media coverage concerning the vaccine, the Catholic Church, and in-school vaccination programs in 2008 was negative. A Canadian Press (2008) story ran on 28 June with the headline, "Premier Scolds Board for Refusing HPV Vaccine." The Halton Catholic District School Board had made the decision to forgo vaccination in their schools, and the article quotes McGuinty as saying, "I'm just going to speak as a parent: I am disappointed with that decision." Shortly thereafter, on 5 and

6 June, respectively, the *Globe and Mail* and the *Toronto Star* published letters to their editors condemning the school board's decision, one of which was penned by a staff member of the University Health Network in Toronto (Berman 2008; Robbins 2008). The Halton board's decision resulted in a flurry of media activity, most of it advocating in favour of vaccination in all Ontario schools and criticizing the Catholic board for what was perceived as a linkage between the vaccine and the promotion of pre-marital sex for girls (Berman 2008).

Significant coverage supporting the vaccine beyond the issue of Catholic schools consisted of "endorsement," both by reporters and medical professionals and/or the manufacturer. For example, Branswell (2008) wrote an article published by the *Globe and Mail* discussing the findings of a research paper that demonstrated that having just one sexual partner could put women at risk for HPV infection. She summarizes: "Three years into those partnerships, nearly 50 per cent had been infected at least once." Branswell ends her article by quoting Monika Naus, director of the immunization program at the British Columbia Centre for Disease Control in Vancouver, who said, "The new findings underscore the wisdom of offering HPV vaccine to girls before they have begun to have sex ... you shouldn't wait until you have had one or two partners before you consider HPV vaccine, because there is a risk even with that first partner." Andre Picard (2008), in an article also published in the *Globe and Mail* on 21 October, lauds Harald zur Hausen, the scientist who won the Nobel Prize for discovering which HPV strains cause cervical cancer and genital warts. Picard puts several questions to zur Hausen, which not only explore the significance of his discovery but also its linkage to vaccine development. When asked about the low uptake of the vaccine in Canada (around 50 per cent), zur Hauzen responds, "There needs to be more effective public health information. If there was a better understanding of the benefits, acceptance would be better. Communication is a major problem in this field. And let me be clear: I have no financial relationship with these companies. I make no money from the vaccine. I am speaking freely as a scientist."

In other instances, a direct relationship with the manufacturer existed. The *Edmonton Journal* published a letter to the editor written by James Mansi (2008), the director of medical and scientific affairs of Merck Frosst Canada, wherein Mansi pressed to establish the safety of the vaccine. "According to the Public Health Agency of Canada," he wrote, "the reporting rate for adverse events for Gardasil in Canada is roughly 33 per 100,000 doses distributed. Reports are mostly of minor adverse events. This is comparable to the rate of reported adverse events for all vaccines in Canada, which has varied from 16 to 40 per 100,000 doses over the period 1992–2004." The letter then listed government agencies and medical societies who had publicly endorsed the vaccine, including the NACI, the Regroupement des Gynécologues Oncologues du Québec (RGOQ), the SOGC, the GOC, the Society of Canadian Colposcopists (SCC), and the Canadian Paediatric Society. There was, however, no mention of the funding Merck Frosst allocates to medical societies in the form of grants, including the $1.5 million informational grant allocated to the SOGC, which is discussed in chapter 5. Accordingly, medical professionals also wrote into national media outlets to endorse the vaccine in 2008. Letters appeared from physicians in the *National Post* (Shafran 2008), the *Globe and Mail* (Peirson 2008), and the *Toronto Star* (Murphy 2008) encouraging readers to consider the benefits of the vaccine. To offer one example: Murphy (2008) states, "As a gynaecological oncologist who treats cervical cancer patients every day, it is very encouraging to see the provincial government taking a proactive stance on this issue … Despite some negative press about side effects stemming from the HPV vaccine, the frequency of these side effects is rare, and I am a firm believer that the benefits outweigh the risks." The remaining articles analysed for 2008 were neutral in tone. These primarily included articles outlining provincial and territorial school-based vaccination programs rolling out that year.

As the above summary of 2008 articles indicates, the national media coverage was conflicting, divergent, and confusing for readers tasked with making decisions surrounding the HPV vaccine. It is clear that media discourses surrounding potential vaccine risks were gaining traction. It should be noted, however, that the variability in coverage content and tone, as well as the myriad positions on the vaccine, is fairly typical of an emerging technology. As members of the media work through the perceived advantages and disadvantages of a new technology, consensus is hard to find.

Addressing Vaccine Risks, Advocating for Gender Parity, and the Catholic School Controversy Continues (2009–10)

Media coverage in 2009 saw a precipitous decline from the previous two years, with only thirty-nine applicable articles uncovered in my search. Of these, 56 per cent were deemed positive, 9 per cent negative, and 20 per cent as neutral in tone. As the percentage of positive articles increased in 2009, we will start there. Three themes predominated: (1) that the vaccine is safe, and that vaccine benefits outweigh risks when it comes to fighting cancer; (2) that boys should be inoculated alongside girls in school-based programs; and (3) that Catholic schools should indeed offer the vaccine. James Mansi (2009), the regional director of Medical Affairs Canada, again wrote a letter declaring the safety of the vaccine, this one published in the *National Post*, touting the benefits of the vaccine. Andre Picard (2009), a journalist for the *Globe and Mail*, highlighted the rise of cancer in teens and young adults, and an article that appeared in the *Hamilton Spectator* on 20 August, "Gardasil's 'Benefits Still Outweigh the Risks'" (Rabin 2009), referred to the results of a study published in the *Journal of the American Medical Association* (*JAMA*), which concluded the same thing (see Slade et al. 2009). Six letters to the editor published in papers in Western Canada denounced the refusal of some Catholic schools to offer the vaccine, expressing concern at the Church's perceived effort to treat women "as mere chattel to be controlled" (Lieber 2009). The *Edmonton Journal* (Canwest News Service 2009) and the *Calgary Herald* (Zuliani 2009) also ran positive stories favouring the vaccine and its extension to boys in school-based programs.

Negative coverage continued to focus on vaccine risks and efficacy. One particular article, headlined "First, Do No Harm; Those Who Question the Safety of Vaccines are Being Unfairly Attacked," exemplifies this trend. Solomon (2009) writes:

Peer-reviewed vaccination studies, because they tend to be funded by the pharmaceutical industry, are suspect. The pro-vaccine bias of government funding agencies gives short shift to studies proposed by skeptics. Even when dissenting peer-reviewed studies do somehow get funded and published, including in prestigious scientific journals, the studies tend to be dismissed and the authors personally attacked.

Neutral coverage primarily focused upon Merck Frosst's Food and Drug Administration (FDA) application for approval to use Gardasil in males under twenty-six years of age (Sicoli 2009) and low uptake rates of the vaccine across the country (except Quebec) (Graveland 2009).

In 2010, only eleven articles in the national media matched the search criteria. Of those, 90 per cent were positive and 10 per cent were neutral. No negative articles appeared that year. The trend of positive articles by medical professionals endorsing the vaccine continued. For example, two articles in the *Globe and Mail* by Andre Picard published in the same week highlighted the Federation of Medical Women of Canada's position that "boys and men play an important role in the transmission of HPV and that they also suffer from a significant number of HPV-related cancers" (Picard 2010a; see also Picard 2010b). The Federation was not only endorsing the vaccine but also lobbying for the inclusion of boys and men in a publicly funded program. Details of the Federation's lobbying efforts to de-gender the vaccine are covered in chapter 6.

De-gendering Vaccine Coverage Normalized and Questioning the HPV Vaccine Framed as "Anti-science" (2011–14)

Throughout 2011–14, coverage of the vaccine dropped considerably, and positive vaccine coverage became normalized. This coverage focused on low vaccine uptake rates and urged for greater participation in school-based campaigns and the de-gendering of the vaccine in school-based programs. By 2014, we begin to see some foreshadowing of what is to come, with a shift towards a narrative that begins to frame questioning the HPV vaccine as "anti-science."

In 2011, twenty-two related articles appeared in the search and, of these, 90 per cent were positive. These stories focused on the gender angle as well as reports of an increase in oral and anal cancers, calling for wider uptake of the vaccine to prevent these types of cancer. These themes are exemplified by reports in the *Globe and Mail*, by the Canadian Press, and on *Canada AM*. The article appearing in the *Globe and Mail* on 23 October refers to a recommendation by the US Advisory Committee on Immunization Practices (ACIP) that boys be vaccinated due to the spread of the virus through heterosexual sex. The article states that although Health Canada approved the vaccine for use in boys and young men, "few provinces have considered extending the school-based HPV vaccination program to boys" (Stobbe 2011). The article goes on to state, "Some feel it's unlikely that most families will agree to get their sons vaccinated primarily to protect girls." Although the article mentions the role of HPV in genital warts and anal cancer, those interviewed did not feel that these potential health threats would mobilize people. The *Canada AM* piece features an interview with prominent health journalist and physician Dr. Marla Shapiro, who attempts to de-gender the HPV vaccine. Shapiro states, "We are recommending universal immunization. In Canada we have had permission to use the quadrivalent vaccine in boys for the past year and a half or so … [I]t's important for us to recognize that HPV is not a gender-based disease" (Canada AM 2011). An endorsement by a physician had not been seen in media coverage since the introduction of the vaccine, and perhaps never by one with such a prominent profile in the Canadian media. And finally, for 2011, a Canadian Press story highlighted the link between HPV and mouth and throat cancers because of the "prevalence of oral sex" (Blatchford 2011).

Media coverage increased slightly in 2012, with thirty-four suitable articles appearing in the search. As in 2011, the stories in 2012 were overwhelmingly positive, at 71 per cent. Only 17 per cent of stories presented a negative bent, and 11 per cent were neutral in tone. The positive coverage centred on the announcement of Ontario's catch-up programming for girls who did not receive the vaccine during middle school, thus extending subsidized coverage to grade 12. This announcement was framed in terms of equity, highlighting that the vaccine would be offered for free to a larger group of girls at public health clinics. The City of Toronto's associate medical officer of health stated, "We hope that as the word gets out and as people realize that it's a safe vaccine and important to prevent cervical cancer – and it would otherwise be expensive if they had to buy it on their own – that they'll come to our clinic and get it" (Canadian Press 2012). The positive coverage also featured several physician endorsements, including ones by the Canadian Medical Association at their annual general meeting, by individual doctors in letters to editors (e.g., Pellizzari 2012), and by doctors in question and answer sessions about the vaccine (Donohue and Roach 2012). Pellizzari (2012) made the following appeal:

> If protecting one's children from cancer isn't enough motivation, perhaps knowing that HPV is independently associated with an increase in HIV acquisition may tip the scales in favour of vaccination. This virus is both pervasive and certain strains of it are deadly. So, although public health nurses will be offering free HPV vaccine in schools for grade 8 girls it is my advice that ALL parents of ALL children aged nine years or older should be giving this vaccination serious consideration.

The remainder of the positive coverage lauded the Calgary Catholic School District's decision to allow the HPV vaccine in their schools, a reversal of an earlier ban. A *Globe and Mail* article stated that the "HPV vaccine has long been seen as controversial because critics, including leaders of the Catholic Church, argued that it would promote promiscuity," and applauded the change as "long overdue, according to a large number of health experts and advocates" (Weeks 2012). The positive media coverage of this decision ran in contrast to negative coverage of the vaccine instigated by Catholic officials in Calgary. These arguments centred on the twin beliefs that the vaccine has no place in Catholic schools because it is not congruent with Catholic faith and doctrine, which promotes abstinence and a restrained morality, and that the vaccine is too new to ascertain its efficacy and safety. Carly Weeks's coverage of the ban reversal appears to play into stereotypes that Catholic viewpoints on sexual activity are a primary concern of the Church and are homogenous to the point of excluding their concerns, such as the validity of the short-term data surrounding the vaccine. As Bishop Fred Henry (2012) of Calgary stated,

> For Catholics, there is no such thing as a purely "health" issue. All activities proposed for a Catholic school need to be assessed in light of our faith and doctrine. This is self-evidently necessary in the case of a vaccine against a disease that is transmitted by sexual activity, which impacts not only the physical, but also the spiritual, psychological and moral well-being of an individual.

In another article published a few months later, Bishop Henry further stated, "The only winner in all of this is Merck, who are probably going to make another ton of money on exaggerated claims based on incomplete and limited scientific data and on our fear of cancer" (quoted in Schneider 2012).

In terms of neutral coverage, articles continued the trend of reporting on low uptake rates. A *Globe and Mail* article cited "as many as 30 to 40 per cent of eligible Canadian girls not being immunized against sexually transmitted disease," with parents fearing "not having enough information about the vaccine, feeling rushed to make a decision about whether their children should get it, and questions about its safety" (Leung 2012).

In 2013, similar media coverage appeared. Of twenty-six relevant articles, 96 per cent were positive. These focused on de-gendering the vaccine, which largely coincided with the decision of the provincial governments of Prince Edward Island and Alberta to vaccinate boys. This positive coverage may have been spurred on by SOGC media advocacy. The organization's then CEO, Dr. Jennifer Blake, wrote to ministers of health across the country urging them to follow PEI's lead in "opening up its program to both genders" (Branswell 2013a). Other positive coverage centred on research that suggested moving from three doses to two, which would be less expensive for provincial governments (Branswell 2013b). The lone negative story in 2013 highlighted, unsurprisingly, the potential safety risks of the vaccine, a persistent theme amongst opponents.

In 2014, only twenty-five articles appeared in the search, with 88 per cent deemed positive, 4 per cent negative, and 8 per cent neutral. Much of the positive coverage focused on issues of SOGC endorsement of the vaccine in an effort to prevent cervical cancer (Gabriel 2014), the increase in HPV-related cancers (Kirkey 2014), and the need for boys to be vaccinated in subsidized, school-based programs (*Montreal Gazette* 2014). Most of the remaining positive coverage appeared as a critique of

Catholic schools, with Weeks (2014) reporting in the *Globe and Mail* on a large-scale study that found that "vaccinating girls against ... HPV ... doesn't lead them to rush out and have sex." Where some people were critical of this research for seeming self-evident, Weeks defends that "a surprising number of people continue to ignore some very basic realities about science and instead erroneously frame the debate about public vaccination as a moral quandary." Weeks's article follows a familiar dichotomous pattern in HPV vaccine reporting: right versus wrong, science versus religion, and, ultimately, rationality versus irrationality. In this type of reporting, questioning the vaccine becomes tantamount to questioning "science." For example, Weeks positions the perspective of Del Grande (then chair of the Toronto Catholic School Board who argued that supporting the vaccine resulted in Christians giving in to secularization) as irrational in the following quote:

> It is a slap in the face to science – instead of celebrating the fact that we now have access to a shot that can prevent the majority of cervical cancer cases, some people are caught up in a patronizing debate over whether allowing access to this medical breakthrough will corrupt the morals of the nation's young girls.

The phrase "a slap in the face to science" undermines the notion that the HPV vaccine could present a "quandary" of any sort, casting objections to it as baseless and dangerous. The tone of Weeks's article sets the stage for the significant media battle surrounding the vaccine that occurred in early 2015.

Public Health and Media "Showdown" over HPV Vaccine Safety and Academic Regulation of "Anti-vaccine" Research (2015–16)

The 2015–16 period was punctuated by two distinct events that shut down alternative narratives to the swell of positive media coverage that had been building over the years: the *Toronto Star* and public health showdown, as well as the withdrawal of an article in the academic journal *Vaccine* for faulty science. Media coverage in 2015 was of a volume on par with that in 2007 due to a "showdown" between media outlets and public health and physician groups over potential vaccine risks. This began on 5 February with the *Toronto Star*'s front-page story, "A Wonder Drug's Dark Side." This discussion of the potential risks associated with the vaccine featured stories of several young women who claimed to have suffered side effects. A public health backlash ensued. The benefits and harms of this article were debated in the *Toronto Star* for the next two weeks, including Heather Mallick's article on 6 February, "Vaccine Debate Is One We Shouldn't Even Be Having." Mallick (2015) opens by stating that the article published the day before

> was about information, and access to it. It was not about the drug itself – it is safe and effective – but about parents and girls not always being told what they need to know in order to make informed decisions, and being dismissed by doctors when they became terribly ill.

An editorial in the same vein also ran echoing that while the vaccine is safe, the public has the right to make informed decisions. This, the editorial suggests, is responsible journalism. The editorial reads as follows:

> The benefits of the popular HPV vaccine Gardasil are well-documented … Still, no drug is without risks. And a *Star* investigation this week shows that risks associated with Gardasil may not be being clearly communicated by health officials to girls receiving the vaccine – or their parents … [S]ince 2008, 60 girls and women in Canada have convulsed or developed disabling joint and muscle pain and other debilitating conditions after receiving Gardasil. (It is not known if the conditions were caused by the drug.) This is not to take anything away from the benefits of the HPV vaccine, or its safety record. Nor is it to suggest the forward-thinking programs in schools to vaccinate young girls against the virus should be halted … That being said, whenever a drug is being prescribed patients have the right to know of any possible side-effects or risks. (*Toronto Star* 2015a)

This balanced journalistic tone came to a halt on 11 February with an article written by Juliet Guichon and Rupert Kaul and supported by sixty-three specialists in infectious disease, public health, and related sciences. In "Science Shows HPV Vaccine Has No Dark Side," Guichon and Kaul (2015) write:

> Given the power of HPV vaccine to prevent disease and death, a long *Toronto Star* article [with] its litany of horror stories and its innuendo give the incorrect impression that the vaccine caused harm … Very unfortunately, this article may well lead readers to doubt both the scientific evidence and the recommendations of the Public Health Agency of Canada.

Guichon and Kaul paint the *Toronto Star* article of 5 February as causing "fear" and not being founded in science. The "balanced" journalistic approach the *Toronto Star* touted as integral shifts further with a piece on 13 February from the paper's public editor, Kathy English (2015), who writes:

"As with many of our other articles published as part of our ongoing investigation into drug safety, this one is mainly about transparency. In this case, transparency for girls and their parents so that they get all of the available risk and benefit information," the reporters stated last week. That's a valid intent but unfortunately, I don't think that's what came through to a great many readers – hence the intense public outcry ... In its overall presentation, the *Star* provided mixed messages. It needed to make crystal clear ... that the scientific evidence has concluded the vaccine is safe and that there is no evidence at all to indicate that the ill effects the young women reported ... were caused by the vaccine.

And in a letter to the editor on 14 February, Dr. Ronald Gold (2015) states that the original article "unwittingly supports the anti-vaccination movement by providing yet more anecdotes of suffering attributed to human papillomavirus (HPV) vaccine." Commentary like this from the medical community led the *Toronto Star* to permanently remove the original story from its website, with the publisher explaining, "We have concluded that in this case our story treatment led to confusion between anecdotes and evidence" (*Toronto Star* 2015b).

Of the fifty-nine articles identified for 2015, including those from the *Toronto Star* mentioned above, 92 per cent were categorized as positive and covered, primarily, the topic of opening up school-based, subsidized vaccinations to boys across the country (see Branswell 2015; Canadian Press 2015b; *National Post* 2015). The five negative articles in 2015 centred on a BC Catholic bishop who argued that abstinence was a better prevention method than the vaccine (see Canadian Press 2015a). The issue of opening up the HPV vaccine to boys was also the dominant theme in the 2016 coverage (see Ferguson 2016; Canadian Press 2016b).

In the first six months of 2016, nineteen articles were identified, with 95 per cent deemed positive. The lone dissenting article published during this time is notable for the controversy that ensued. A small-town BC news site, the *Invermere Valley Echo*, published an editorial by Nicole Trigg on 9 March entitled, "Resistance When Going against the Status Quo." Trigg (2016) questions the removal of an article by two University of British Columbia researchers from the academic journal *Vaccine*; the journal withdrew the article due to "questionable methodology" used to conclude that the vaccine may not be safe. Trigg posited that *Vaccine* had succumbed to pharmaceutical interests, concluding, "In its Gardasil warning, the American College of Pediatricians stated it's committed to the prevention of disease by vaccines, but this didn't stop it from declaring further Gardasil studies were warranted. As these new studies emerge that contradict the status quo, the pro-anti-vaccine debate can't be allowed to drown out the voice of reason." This editorial was preceded by a *National Post* article on 18 February, which reported that "Canadian scientists – heavily funded by anti-vaccination foundations – say their latest study may have been pulled because of pressure from pharmaceutical companies or governments un-happy with their findings" (Blackwell 2016b). Blackwell quotes one of those scientists as saying that "sound research is being suppressed and (the) pharma-lobby has spread everywhere their propaganda like metas-tases." When the article was "permanently withdrawn," Blackwell (2016a) wrote further, revealing that the editor of *Vaccine* had worked previously for Merck Frosst, the vaccine's manufacturer.

Conclusion

HPV vaccine news coverage in Canada over the near-decade from 2007 to mid-2016 followed a definitive arc that, when examined closely, re-veals a narrative that has been shaped by a communications program, outlined in chapters 5 and 6, that allowed a pharmaceutical company to put into place its sales/governance strategies (see Figure 1). This story arc initially relied heavily on the notion of the "risky girl/woman," and then eventually extended this leitmotif to all genders. It began with a heavy-handed depiction of the threat of cervical cancer, which was then temporarily interrupted by the "What's the hurry?" narrative thread. This thread did not discount the potential benefits of the vaccine but rather urged for more research to be conducted before a national school-based immunization program roll-out. This initial story arc was followed by a period, from 2008 to 2010, when potential vaccine risk, due to the lack of long-term research, dominated media discussions surrounding the vaccine. This was then followed, finally, by a repositioning of HPV vaccine coverage, which started to normalize the vaccine and generate overwhelmingly positive reportage.

This shift in narrative was not incidental. There was a concerted effort on behalf of the pharmaceutical company Merck Frosst to fill media cov-erage with physician endorsements (an offshoot of the position statements released by medical societies), position statements, and policy papers. This communications strategy is often not covered in the anthropology of policy research, nor in critical public policy research, but is an elemental compo-nent of any sales/governance strategy. These strategies are multi-pronged and discursive, and they are employed along Foucault's (1991) descrip-tion of power apparatuses, which are distributed in a net-like fashion. This is how these discourses take such strong hold, creating "truths" that are pervasive, surrounding us through advertising, governmental programs, and everyday media coverage. The positive media coverage of the vaccine, which started to take hold in 2008, became solidly normalized between

Figure 1. Media coverage themes from 2007 through 2016

2007
Gendered Framing
Endorsement Coverage
"What's the Hurry?"

2008
Endorsement Coverage Continues
Vaccine Risks (Potential Side Effects)
Catholic School Board Refuses Vaccination
Catholic Bishops' Opposition to Vaccine
Expanding Vaccine Indications

2009–2010
Endorsement Coverage Continues
Vaccine Benefits Outweigh Risks
Boys Should Also Be Vaccinated in School Programs
Catholic Schools Should Offer Vaccine

2011–2014
Beginnings of Questioning Vaccine as "Anti-Science"
Positve Coverage Normalized
De-gendered Vaccine in Policy
Low Vaccine Uptake Rates

2015–2016
Shutdown of Counter-Narratives
Endorsement Coverage Continues
Lack of Informed Consent

2011 and 2014, to the extent that critiques of the vaccine were framed as "anti-science." This tactic of positioning even mild critiques about the vaccine as "anti-science" leaves little space for anyone to pose questions without being portrayed as radical or as not acting in the best interests of public health. This narrowing of acceptable discourse sets the stage for the public health condemnation of those deemed "anti-vaxxers."

While this book is not questioning the safety or efficacy of the HPV vaccine, the stakeholder influence on policy development and how women negotiated and made decisions within the confines of this policy, and the silencing of a certain narrative, up to and including lobbying for the permanent removal of news coverage while actively promoting a competing narrative, is a troubling trend in Canadian journalism. This begs the question of whether or not pharmaceutical companies' indirect lobbying is, in part, responsible for the narrowing of media discourse surrounding vaccines. It is in such an environment that Canadian women must assess information in order to make HPV vaccination decisions for themselves and their children.

5 Vaccine Marketing by Harnessing Hegemonic Cultural Discourses of Risk and Gender

Introduction

In introducing the HPV vaccine to North American markets, Merck Frosst employed a gender-based approach to marketing, which leverages hegemonic cultural logics concerning gender and health risk and functions as a sales/governance strategy that places girls/women in a predetermined box removed from sites of power. In order to keep girls/women in this box, the HPV vaccine is positioned as a cancer fighting mechanism. This sidesteps HPV as a sexually transmitted infection (STI) and proffers a vast platform for sales/governance because cancer, as opposed to STIs, is culturally interpreted as wide-reaching, mysterious, fear inducing, and multi-causal. This framing was picked up by Merck Frosst's stakeholder ally, the Society of Obstetricians and Gynaecologists of Canada (SOGC), in successive campaigns, from the introduction of the vaccine to the present day. The SOGC maintained the gendered framing of the HPV vaccine well past its approval for vaccinating boys and men in Canada, and this framing persists, despite boys now being folded in school-based vaccination programs across the country. I argue that the SOGC has continued to brand HPV as a "women's issue" and has contributed to the persistence of HPV and the HPV vaccine being viewed as predominantly relevant to girls and women. As such, the SOGC continues to contribute to the deployment of gender as risk.

Merck Frosst's Gender-Based Marketing

Why is there an emphasis on vaccinating women in introductory policy documents? In other words, why was HPV so clearly gendered in public health programming for nearly ten years? The answers to these questions lie in the roll-out strategy for the vaccine developed by Merck Frosst and deployed simultaneously by medical societies in Canada, which lead public health policymaking in an environment where there is little existing research on the prevalence of HPV or an awareness of or knowledge about HPV. The Gardasil roll-out strategy had a three-pronged approach: (1) release the vaccine for nine- to twenty-six-year-old girls and women; (2) focus on women aged twenty-six to forty-five; and (3) make it available to boys and men (Hersko-vits 2007, 70). Each phase of the strategy hinged upon gender-based analyses: gender cohorts were researched exhaustively and made the target of each section of the marketing campaign in a common current tactic called "segmented marketing" (Sheth, Sisodia, and Sharma 2000). Merck Frosst's marketing campaign depended on the gendering of HPV and the positioning of Gardasil as a cancer-fighting mechanism for women, sidestepping the issue of sexual health and related cancers in other genders. In 2007, the magazine *Pharmaceutical Executive* awarded Merck Frosst its first "Brand of the Year" award for the Gardasil campaign.

Pharmaceutical Executive describes the marketing campaign as "play[ing] on cancer fears, but [drawing] on themes of safeguarding your children (for moms) and empowerment (for girls)" (Herskovits 2007, 68). Merck Frosst conceived of and delivered a two-part advertising campaign. The first part, "Make the Connection," appeared prior to the approval of the vaccine and was intended to increase awareness of HPV. The second phase, post-approval, was a branding effort called "Tell Someone." It was intended to "tap into 'women's natural inclination' as talkers and sharers" according to the Merck Frosst vice-president assigned the Gardasil portfolio (Herskovits 2007, 68). The "Tell Someone" campaign evolved into the two types of Gardasil advertisements that are still circulating in Canada today: those targeting young women of university age (through television, magazines, large banners at university student centres, university-sponsored day planners, and posters in university washroom stalls); and those targeting the mothers of girls near the grade 8 vaccination age and the girls themselves (through television and women's magazines). The "mom" campaign works to specifically support Ontario's official in-school HPV vaccination program. As the Ontario government rolled out the school-based vaccination campaign, it did not initiate a public information campaign concerning HPV or the vaccine. Merck Frosst marketing campaigns filled that gap. This marketing campaign consists of information pamphlets, print advertisements (as described in the preceding chapter on mothers and their decision-making for their daughters), and commercials.

Sales/Governance Strategies

How can a pharmaceutical branding campaign gender a virus and sub-sequent public health programming? It is not simply that the multina-tional pharmaceutical corporation with the most dollars or persuasive lobbyists triumphs, even though direct and indirect lobbying activities were both numerous and expensive, as is detailed in chapter 6. Rather, the situation is more complex; economic power is embedded in, and not above, social, cultural, and historical processes (Morrison 1995, 320). In this specific case, Merck Frosst strategically harnessed Western hegem-onic cultural logics and discourses surrounding risk and gender in order to develop marketing campaigns to sell its vaccine. This was a two-part process that involved (1) circulating HPV-related information that lever-aged cultural logics surrounding risk and gender in order to brand HPV as a woman-only concern; and (2) arranging consumer buy-in through self-regulation. The first step was to disseminate HPV-related "expert knowledge" (Foucault 1989, 52–61). As publicly available government information on the vaccine was limited, Merck Frosst readily filled this void. Merck Frosst used the advertorial "Make the Connection" cam-paign to inform women about HPV. It contains information on cervical cancer, what HPV is, and the many different HPV strains. This informa-tion is supported by statistics of the global incidence of cervical cancer, an anatomical drawing of a woman's reproductive system and endorse-ments provided by leaders in the field of women's health in the United States. While this is a paid advertisement, it reads and looks as though it is a medical information brochure.

These pamphlets were followed by the "Tell Someone" commercials. An example of such a commercial features two women – a middle-aged physician in a white coat with a stethoscope and a woman in her mid-thirties wearing a casual T-shirt with her hair partially pulled back. As the name of the commercial indicates, the women are featured discussing how serious cervical cancer is and how as women – both as a female phy-sician and an "ordinary" woman – they have a duty to tell other women about HPV, its commonality, and that it is a causal factor of cervical can-cer. These pamphlets and commercials can still be found on the internet today, in 2023, by conducting a Google or YouTube search.

It is important to note that these "Make the Connection" and "Tell Someone" campaigns were developed and released prior to the approval of Gardasil by the Food and Drug Administration (FDA) in the United States. Because of this, Merck Frosst was not able to mention the Gardasil vaccine by name in its advertisements. The next wave of Gardasil adver-tising, post-FDA approval, depicts a mother and a daughter, urging the mother to talk to her doctor about her daughter's vaccination. The information about HPV provided in the pre-approval advertisements and the push to get women vaccinated in the post-approval advertisements work together to scare women about HPV and to create a "need" for inoculation against HPV.

The second step involved getting consumer buy-in, literally. Merck Frosst created such a need for the vaccine in its multiple advertising campaigns that consumers asked their doctors for it. This is a common tactic of pharmaceutical companies and is called direct-to-consumer advertising (Mintzes 2010). This tactic is essentially pharmaceutically directed self-regulation. As such, Gardasil sales tactics also function as governance strategies. Such a governance approach works to deploy "a mode of power par excellence designed to produce a market-based notion of agency and subjectivity" (Giroux 2010, 30). To critique this governance strategy, I am employing Foucault's (1991) concept of governmentality. The governmentality approach to risk focuses on how governments "work together to govern – that is, manage and regulate – populations via risk discourses and strategies" (Lupton 1999a, 1). Governmentality is not necessarily about governmental institutions, however. Instead, it is about their ability to get those they are governing to enact their policies and directives through "persuasion" (Giroux 2010, 51–2).

Within the current, contemporary climate of "new" public health, which emphasizes neo-liberal devolution of governmental responsibility (Lupton and Petersen 1996), governing approaches focus more and more on "the art of self-government, connected with morality" (Foucault, 1991, 91). Nettleton (1996, 34) calls this the "rise of a psycho-socioenvironmental/ epidemiological model," which has replaced the biomedical approach. This shift results in moving away from treating disease and towards preventing disease. Prevention policy, which is delivered via health promotion strategies, is predicated upon the tenets of "'risk,' 'surveillance,' and the 'rational self'" (Nettleton 1996, 34). As such, preventative strategies, or "technologies of power" (Foucault, 1999, 14), centre on the promotion of self-regulation, which works to attain and maintain an idealized form of self (Turner 1997, xii). Contemporary health discourse focuses on a version of the self "that is autonomous, subjective and active" (Nettleton 1997, 209). In other words, it is up to *you* to ensure that *you* meet the standards of health and to manage any potential health risks. Thus, if a person falls sick, it is due to their lack of self-restraint. Idealized conceptualizations of the self are then steeped in the notions of self-discipline and the ability to continually reinforce an identity that promotes one's health.

All individuals are expected to be "active citizens," whether or not they are actually part of "targeted populations" (Dean 1999, 147), albeit the lines between those who are targeted and those who are not are porous – all can be at risk at any time. This is part and parcel of the "colonization of the future" (Giddens 1991, 117, 182), whereby risk has become a foundational tenet of governance strategies. As such, "it seems that we are no longer simply concerned with the governance *of* risk but we are now in an era of governance *by* risk" (Rothstein 2006, 216; emphasis in original). Governance through pre-detection, or creating what Nikolas Rose (2007, 20) calls "prepatients," opens up increasingly fertile ground for surveillance (Castel 1991, 288). In their work on risk and governmentality, Rose and Carlos Novas (2005) put forth the notion of biological citizenship, in which governmentality is linked to governance via the body. Biological citizenship follows the dominant trend in risk theory literature as it does not critically address gender. As is discussed in chapter 7, "situated risk" (Boholm 2003) provides more fertile ground through which to pursue risk and gender in tandem. Moreover, Henry Giroux (2010, 2) posits that in the current neo-liberal landscape, individuals are organized not "as citizens but as consumers."

The expansive surveillance mandate of the new public health functions by "mainly incorporat[ing] voluntary actions on the part of citizens but also [by] us[ing] legislation, much of which is enshrined in public health acts" (Lupton and Petersen 1996, 5). As seen with the Gardasil campaigns, women are urged to accept greater responsibility for their health through direct-to-consumer advertising. But Gardasil sales are also ensured because of the province-wide grade 8 public school vaccination program for girls in Ontario. As the Government of Ontario did not initiate a public information campaign alongside the grade 8 programming, Merck Frosst's multi-pronged Gardasil advertising campaigns worked to ensure that a need for the vaccine was maintained. In the case of Gardasil, the responsibility for the health of the population was no longer *entirely* under the purview of the state. While the responsibility for keeping risk at bay is that of the individual's, what is deemed to be a risk is established through the joint workings of pharmaceutical companies and policymaking processes. Together they create a guaranteed market for the sale of the product. This would not happen, however, if prevailing cultural logics did not support the notion of women being perpetually at risk.

The Society of Obstetricians and Gynaecologists of Canada Follows Suit with Promotional Campaigns

As is documented by Erin Connel (2010), the SOGC released an early promotional campaign for the vaccine in 2006. The SOGC received a

$1.5 million informational grant from Merck Frosst in order to produce this campaign (Page 2007a), so the similarities are not surprising. This campaign hinged on the website HPVinfo.ca (which still operates today with updated materials) and marketing collaterals, including just under 250,000 magnetic bookmarks, 135,000 brochures, and posters that were meant to be affixed to the back of washroom stall doors in women's bathrooms on university and college campuses across Canada. Additionally, the campaign produced TV commercials that were distributed to eighty stations across Canada, a radio advertisement that was sent to 500 radio stations, and a print campaign aimed at middle school and secondary school teachers in order to support school-based vaccination campaigns and public health catch-up clinics (Connel 2010). In 2006, the SOGC created a brochure aimed at convincing mothers to inoculate their middle school-aged daughters.

From a visual perspective, the SOGC brochure uses large-type for certain words, which are also emboldened in bright, "feminine" colours, including "myths," "cancer," "burden," and "disease," as well as images of mothers caressing or caringly holding their daughters to reinforce the message that girls should be vaccinated against cancer, and that middle-class, well-groomed, and caring mothers are the ones who carry out this act in order to protect their daughters. The campaign website is also featured prominently, encouraging individuals to seek more vaccine information there. The similarities of this brochure to Gardasil's own advertising are striking. The look, messaging, and feel of the Gardasil ads and the SOGC campaign gives the appearance of a coordinated marketing campaign that was orchestrated between the manufacturer and a prominent medical society.

As mentioned above, the website HPVinfo.ca (or infoVPH.ca for the French version) was still in operation at the time of writing this chapter, in 2017, but had expanded its focus to include males and older women in their thirties and forties to reflect the expanded vaccine indications in Canada, while still maintaining its primary focus on the original mandate: middle school-aged girls and their mothers. For example, the then-current SOGC HPV vaccine website featured a photo of two young people holding hands, both dressed in jeans with one individual wearing a metallic belt. The shot was taken from the waist down, so the gender of the individuals was unknown, although one hand had longer nails than the other, implying a heterosexual couple. The tag line across this image read, "Spread the word, not the disease. The facts on human papillomavirus from Canada's experts." This tag line corresponded with the text at the bottom of the page, which stated, "HPVinfo.ca delivers evidence-based information about the human papillomavirus. All material on this site is developed and reviewed by health-care professionals and is based on guidelines from the Society of Obstetricians and Gynaecologists of Canada (SOGC). HPVinfo.ca is administered by the SOGC, Canada's leading authority on sexual and reproductive health." It also featured a band of four photographs: a young man and woman kissing; two teenagers – one male and one female – on their phones; a mother and a teenaged daughter and son; and a smiling teenage girl casually reclining. The majority of those pictured were represented as female, and the next large image below was of a teenaged girl eating from a cereal bowl while reclining on a bed, reading a book. Again, the tagline "Spread the word, not the disease" appeared, this time in a circle graphic to her right. The imaging and messaging from earlier SOGC informational campaigns remained constant.

The SOGC did take a minor detour from its consistent messaging regarding mothers and teenage girls to debut a campaign geared at women between the ages of twenty-five and forty-five in the fall of 2016. While this was a slight divergence in target audience, the vaccine remained gendered in SOGC promotions nonetheless. As per a press release on 7 October 2016, "The incidence of HPV is increasing among women in their 30s and 40s – women who have likely never displayed any symptoms, yet could still become infected with genital warts or cancer. As we age it is more difficult for our bodies to rid ourselves of the virus" (SOGC 2016). The press release also mentioned a "provocative video which is playing at selected Cineplex theatres across Canada over the next two weeks [10–21 October]." The video is still available for viewing on YouTube and is titled "HPV – You Could Be at Risk" (see HealthSOGC 2016). The advertisement features a women in her thirties or forties who appears to be single, as she is perusing a dating website on her laptop computer in her apartment or condo on a dark and stormy night. The voiceover features a women who says the following: "Up to three in four sexually active Canadian will be infected with HPV. It's a virus and it can lead to cancer. Ask your doctor. Visit HPVinfo.ca." The woman featured in the video does not speak, and the advertisement ends with the HPVinfo.ca website address on the screen.

Deploying Gender as Risk

In the case of the HPV vaccine, being a certain gender puts one at risk. As a girl/woman, being female positions you as needing particular protection from cancer stemming from HPV, yet this protection is not deemed necessary for men. Douglas ([1966] 2002, xix) asserts that "arguments about risk are highly charged, morally and politically." As such, the attribution of being at risk for potential illness encourages moral governance through the framing and fixing of difference. This morality is used to keep those who threaten the social order – or the equilibrium of those in power – safely within their predetermined "box" (Douglas [1966] 2002, 125, 172). Douglas ([1966] 2002, 125) refers to "Chinese-box-like" structures, where boxes fit within boxes, each indicating the multiple layers of derivative structures sitting within the overall structure, or the main box, a metaphor for society as a whole. When in a box, those at risk can be contained and governed. When placed within the box, one has to follow the rules or norms. The norm "is not simply and not even a principle of intelligibility; it is an element on the basis of which a certain exercise of power is founded and legitimized … Perhaps we could say it is a political concept" (Foucault 1999, 50). Thus, this at-risk categorization reflects not only women's subordinate status in Western society but also works to maintain this subordination. The cultural messaging surrounding the HPV vaccine, both in the pharmaceutical marketing campaigns and the Ontario government policy of subsidizing in-school vaccination for girls only, works to keep women and girls firmly in their at-risk box. This is a governance strategy to keep women in their place in the social hierarchy – it does not relegate them to the margins but keeps them firmly tucked away from spheres of influence.

There is, of course, a long history of keeping women in their place through their being labelled "at risk." In medicine, as in society, women have been portrayed as "especially threatening to the moral order and social stability of society, largely due to the seemingly uncontrollable and dangerous nature of their sexuality" (Lupton 2003, 143). Douglas ([1966] 2002) elaborates further:

> Such patterns of sexual danger can be seen to express symmetry or hierarchy. It is implausible to interpret them as expressing something about the actual relation of the sexes. I suggest that many ideals about sexual dangers are better interpreted as symbols of relation between parts of society, as mirroring designs of hierarchy or symmetry, which apply in the larger social system. (4)

In other words, positioning women as sexually threatening is not reflective of gender relations – those between men and women within a heterosexual framework – but of society's tendency to classify and find a place for everyone so as to not disturb existing power structures.

Correspondingly, for several hundred years, women have been positioned as the "other" in medicine, unwell and inferior to men (Lupton 2003, 143). Women have been, and continue to be, portrayed as faint-hearted, prone to disease, vessels for spreading sexually transmitted infections, and the cause of emotional turmoil for their children. Medicine has woven the tale that women are both tautologically passive receptors of disease and active, deleterious agents of disease (Lupton 2003, 143). Women are represented as such in medical textbooks. For example, Emily Martin (2007, 417) reports that medical texts depict male and female reproductive organs as "systems of production," but frame male organic matter in an active and positive light, all the while depicting female organic matter in disparaging terms. Sperm is generally described as being "produced," whereas "ova merely sit on the shelf, slowly degenerating and aging like overstocked inventory" (Martin 2007, 418). Sperm is also depicted as "penetrating the egg" through "mechanical and chemical means" after the egg has "drifted along the fallopian tube" (Martin 2007, 420–1). Martin finds that such imagery haunts historical and contemporary representations, even when research has detected new patterns of reproduction. For example, in spite of the discovery by Johns Hopkins scientists that the sperm and egg adhere similarly to positive and negative strips of Velcro, the process is still described using the old imagery. Martin (2007) explains:

> Although this new version of the saga of the egg and the sperm broke through cultural expectations, the researchers who made the discovery continued to write papers and abstracts as if the sperm were the active party who attacks, binds, penetrates, and enters the egg. The only difference was that the sperm were now seen as performing these actions weakly. (421)

Likewise, Susan Lawrence and Kae Bendixen (1992) note that medical textbooks from the late 1890s to the late 1980s depict male and female forms in a similar manner. Anatomical imagery and accompanying text place a primacy on male bodies by using these bodies as the ideal benchmark and then describe female bodies through the ways they differ from the male "standard." These cultural conceptualizations also translate into medical practice. Gynaecology, as a medical specialty, holds no equivalent area of research or service for men, even though men possess their own specific set of genitalia. As such, female genitalia are classified as risky and are subjected to surveillance throughout a woman's life cycle. Barbara Hanson (2000, 60) notes that other potential cancer sites, such as the "liver, pancreas, lymph glands, lung, kidney, or other less accessible organs," are not accorded the same surveillance. Correspondingly, women are routinely screened for breast and cervical cancer due to their unique at-risk status and because these areas are simple to reach (Kaufert 2000). As Hanson (2000, 60) notes, "this opens up the possibility that genitalia focus in cancer may be as much a case of what is routinely screened rather than what is ultimately most dangerous." That being said, gynaecology continues to be a way by which medicine constructs risk in women that cannot be construed in men. Gynaecology keeps women "visible" (Foucault 1989, 111) in medicine and continual "subjects" of surveillance and control (Lupton 2003, 161).

Thus, the sexually active "feminine" body (Bartky 1990) was (and is) viewed as needing to be monitored and sheltered from harm. Protecting oneself is not thought to come "naturally" for the "weaker," second sex. This is, of course, a not very subtle reference to Simone de Beauvoir's (1952) well-known tome. But making genitalia and sexual activity visible is also a long-standing governance technique. Foucault notes that instead of "repressing" the subject of sex, modern power structures amplify it. He urges readers to look at how power functions in "positive mechanisms, insofar as they produce knowledge, multiply discourse, induce pleasure, and generate power" (Foucault [1978] 1990, 73). It is through promoting discussions about sex, sexuality, and gender that power structures are able to make women visible and simultaneously keep them within the box that Douglas ([1966] 2002) speaks of. But with the case of the HPV vaccine, early research based in the United States indicated that parents were not likely to vaccinate their daughters if they felt that the vaccine promoted adolescent sexuality (Constantine and Jerman 2007; Dekker 2006; Olshen et al. 2005). In some studies, parents even described the vaccine as a means of promoting and encouraging adolescent sexuality, a concept with which they were clearly uncomfortable.

Given this research, Merck Frosst did not harness tried-and-true methods of highlighting women's sexual risk or risks relating to sexuality; that is, they did not focus on HPV as an STI. Instead, Merck Frosst chose to frame HPV solely as a cancer-causing virus – one that specifically causes cervical cancer – and sidestepped the fact that HPV is transmitted through sexual contact, including genital touching (Burchell et al. 2011; Vanslyke et al. 2008, 584). Merck Frosst was well aware that positioning the HPV vaccine as a tool to fight STIs in girls/women was not a smart marketing move; in this case, sex would not sell. (Sex, of course, was meant to sell when Merck Frosst introduced an advertising campaign for the use of the vaccine in young men in 2012. This campaign positioned Gardasil as a genital wart fighter for its male customers [Merck Frosst 2011b].) Instead, Merck Frosst developed a strategy to sell the vaccine by playing upon cultural notions of the "female" who needs to be protected from cancer. Mixing the cultural notions of the "weaker" sex that must be protected and cancer as a frightening, mysterious, and omnipresent illness (Sontag 1999) was the perfect marketing prescription. I am not saying that cancer is not a terrible illness for those who suffer from it. Rather, I am pointing to a very specific set of Western cultural notions and logics about cancer that are emotionally charged and that Merck Frosst leveraged in the selling of its vaccine: cancer is feared and not widely understood, most individuals know, or know of, someone who has suffered from cancer, and this is a disease from which all parents wish to protect their children. In Merck Frosst's marketing of the HPV vaccine, cancer kept girls/women visible but sex invisible. Even though this tactic differs slightly from Foucault's summation of visibility and sexual relations, the power technique employed reflects Foucault's ideas. It is also interesting to note that Merck Frosst focused on cervical cancer and not vaginal, vulvar, anal, or throat cancer in women. This is because cervical cancer is an easier cultural sell than the other cancers associated with HPV.

As will be discussed below, the main tenets of Merck Frosst's marketing campaign – the gendering of the vaccine and its positioning as a cancer panacea – spilled over into Canadian public health policymaking. Some might call this the "pharmaceuticalization of public health" (Biehl 2007, 222), but I argue that this is really a case of the replication of hegemonic conceptualizations of gender and risk in policymaking. Merck Frosst was the first to deploy these governance techniques as a selling mechanism, but if these conceptualizations were not in the ether, they would not have been picked up again in policymaking. The policy sphere, as with all other facets of daily life, is rife with the circulating, yet static, cultural "ideals" of gender and risk.

Conclusion

This chapter charts how, through descriptions of the sales/governance strategies employed, Merck Frosst and the Society of Obstetricians and Gynaecologists of Canada pursued gender-based marketing that hinged on the notion of the HPV-related at-risk girl/woman. This gender-based marketing persists today, despite the approval of the HPV vaccine for boys and men and the inclusion of boys in school-based programs across Canada. This gender-based marketing leverages hegemonic cultural logics concerning gender and health risk and has persisted because it functions as a sales/governance strategy that places girls/women in a predetermined box removed from sites of power. In order to keep girls/women in this box, the HPV vaccine is positioned as a cancer-fighting mechanism. This sidesteps HPV as a sexually transmitted infection and proffers a vast platform for sales/governance because cancer, as opposed to sexually transmitted infections, is culturally interpreted as wide-reaching, mysterious, fear inducing, and multi-causal. By maintaining the gender-based marketing and continuing to position the HPV vaccine as a cancer fighter, the need for the vaccine, both in government programs and through individual take-up, is continually reinforced. The persistence of deploying gender as risk in the case of the HPV vaccine is also seen in the extensive media coverage of the vaccine, which was covered in chapter 4. The cultural logics displayed in gender-based policymaking and gender-based marketing also come into relief, and are therefore reinforced, in media coverage of the vaccine. As a result, the media becomes another conduit for Merck Frosst's extensive strategic stakeholder leverage activities, and one begins to wonder where the reach of this pharmaceutical giant ends.

6 Gendered Vaccine Policymaking

Introduction

This chapter outlines stakeholder influence over public health policymaking in Canada, including the role that pharmaceutical manufacturers play in policymaking processes. The impetus for vaccine policy emanates from the pharmaceutical company itself – in this case, Merck Frosst, which engaged in intense direct and indirect lobbying – and is dispersed across a series of selected stakeholders, with medical societies being the primary conduit. All stakeholders initially pushed for a gendered policy vis-à-vis the vaccine, even though HPV is gender blind and HPV infection can lead to cancer across genders. This decision constructed the notion of the girl/woman who is at risk for cervical cancer and positions HPV as a "women's disease." This construction of the at-risk girl/woman is then transposed into public health policymaking through the application of gender-based analysis (GBA) frames on behalf of the federal government, who in 2007 introduced the HPV vaccine for girls and women only. The GBA invoked by the federal government rests on static and homogenous notions of women as a discrete category of risk. While GBA+, which is intended to bring an intersectional lens to gender-based analyses, was introduced in 2013 to the federal government, it does not appear to have been applied to provincial HPV vaccine policy and program development. Today, boys are vaccinated in schools in all provinces across the country, but this policy development was almost ten years in the making, and groups vulnerable to HPV-related cancers are not prioritized in provincial programs. As a result, gender remains the primary axis in GBA+ as it is applied in HPV vaccine programming. Thus, there is much work to do in developing and implementing nuanced policymaking frameworks invoking gender and intersectionality as a category of analysis.

The Federal and Ontario Governments Roll Out the HPV Vaccine

Mass media accounts generally described the introduction of the HPV vaccine to Canada as a swift development (A. Gordon 2009; Gulli 2007; Picard 2007). This was not, however, the case. In 2005, the Public Health Agency of Canada (PHAC) released a report entitled *Canadian Human Papillomavirus Vaccine Research Priorities Workshop* (the workshop took place 17–18 November of that year). The aim of this workshop was to "examine the current Canadian and international status of HPV vaccine research and develop national research priorities before the vaccines become approved for use in Canada" (PHAC 2005, iii). When referring to vaccines, the report referenced both Gardasil and Cervarix, but Gardasil received approval in July of 2006 for girls/women, whereas Cervarix did not receive such approval until February of 2010 (Health Canada 2006; Picard 2010a, 2010b). At the outset, the workshop report discusses HPV as being connected to multiple genders, but most of the document's text positions HPV as a "women's issue." This is selective framing, as HPV presents in women, men, intersex, and transgender individuals and is linked to both gender-specific and gender-blind cancers (Parkin and Bray 2006). Individuals with male sexual organs can develop penile cancer, and those with female genitalia can develop cervical, vaginal, and vulvar cancers; any gender can develop oropharyngeal (throat) or anal cancer from HPV, as well as HPV-related genital warts and recurrent respiratory papillomatosis, which present as warts in the throat region (Centers for Disease Control and Prevention 2012). However, the PHAC report emphasizes the utility of HPV vaccines in primarily preventing cervical cancer.

Attendees of the November workshop included senior federal bureaucrats, scientists, researchers, physicians, and numerous representatives from Merck Frosst and GlaxoSmithKline Biologicals (PHAC 2005, 28–30). Thus, pharmaceutical companies were present "at the table," even before Merck Frosst officially submitted its request for Health Canada approval of Gardasil on 12 December 2005. It could be argued that the presence of pharmaceutical companies at the governmental planning workshop is a conflict of interest, but their presence should not be surprising considering the current era of what the federal government calls "smart regulation" (Graham 2005). Industry now plays a significant role in governmental regulation processes, from initial consultations regarding the introduction of a product to Canada to its regulatory approval and eventual roll-out. Smart regulation was introduced in March 2005 with the aim to "restructure Canada's regulatory policy … [to] streamline and speed up approval for new drugs, foods, biotechnology products,

veterinary products and pesticides" (Graham 2005, 1469). Smart regulation is geared, simultaneously, to expediting the integration of new
business ventures into the Canadian marketplace and safeguarding the
public interest through strong regulatory frameworks. Janice Graham
(2005, 1469) is sceptical that the government is able to meet these dual
priorities and posits that business interests generally trump those of public health. Within smart regulation frameworks, pharmaceutical companies pay user fees in order to have their drugs reviewed by Health
Canada's Pharmaceutical Drugs Directorate (formerly the Therapeutic
Products Directorate). As Lexchin (1999, 173) observed many years ago,
"as funding for the operations of [this agency] shifts from the government to the drug companies, a situation is created in which the drug
companies could be perceived to be setting the priorities." User fees are
a "cost-recovery" measure. For example, in 2004, 51 per cent of the Directorate's budget came from user fees; the remaining was sourced from
government monies (Silversides 2010, 136). Merck Frosst's application
was processed in seven months due to its application being given priority
review status (Health Canada 2006). It is not surprising that Gardasil
received expedited approval from the Directorate given this regulatory
climate.

On 15 February 2007, the National Advisory Committee on Immunization (NACI) released a report on the HPV vaccine (see NACI 2007).
This was a crucial document in determining the roll-out of the vaccine
because NACI is charged with providing physician recommendations regarding who should be vaccinated and when, and how vaccines should
be administered. This document is exhaustive and references HPV infections in women and men, but primarily focuses on the linkage between
HPV and cervical cancer. The NACI report was publicly released before
the Health Canada Summary Basis of Decision on the vaccine was issued in March 2007. A Summary Basis of Decision document provides
approval for a pharmaceutical to be used in Canada, whereas NACI is
charged with recommending how a vaccine should be utilized. Thus,
the document providing the framework of how a vaccine should be administered was distributed before the vaccine was approved for use in
Canada. Interestingly, the Summary Basis of Decision mentions that boys
aged nine to fifteen had been included in Gardasil clinical trials, but that
research was ongoing in boys and men from sixteen to twenty-six years of
age (Health Canada 2007).

On 27 March 2007, the *Canadian Medical Association Journal* (*CMAJ*)
published a "think piece" in its news section titled, "Debate Begins over
Public Funding for HPV Vaccine." Given the amount of sensationalized
writing that has circulated in the last fifteen years since the approval of

the vaccine in Canada (these media discourses are discussed in chapter 4), this was a thoughtful and balanced article that outlined the potential benefits of the vaccine and potential objections to a public inoculation campaign. The piece also discusses vaccinating boys but mentions that "publicly funded programs are not expected for several years" (Comeau 2007, 913). The *CMAJ* could not have been more wrong. Soon after the NACI report was issued, the Conservative government announced, as part of its April 2007 annual budget, that $300 million would be funnelled on a per capita basis to the provinces and territories "to help establish a national vaccine program that will help protect women and girls from cancer of the cervix" (Department of Finance 2007). This press release positioned HPV and the HPV vaccine strictly as a women's-only issue.

In early August 2007, the Ontario government followed suit and announced it would offer the HPV vaccine to grade 8 girls enrolled in the public school system, free of charge. In its official announcement, the provincial government proclaimed, "we're providing this vaccine to women at a young age so we can help prevent the spread of HPV and save lives" (Office of the Premier 2007). There is no mention in this release of HPV in connection with other genders or cancers, nor the part they play in the transmission of the virus. Ontario followed the federal government's lead in promoting the vaccine for use on girls/women only and as a means to "save" them from cancer. Premier Dalton McGuinty made the announcement in the lobby of Women's College Hospital in Toronto, flanked by female physicians in lab coats. The Government of Ontario's public health program to provide vaccinations to grade 8 girls in school settings is ongoing, although initial participation was tepid. For example, 40 per cent of girls in Toronto did not receive the vaccination when it was offered to them in grade 8, and so in early September 2012, Toronto Public Health announced that it would be delivering free vaccinations to teenage girls aged fourteen to nineteen. The Ontario government agreed to provide the funding for this (Canadian Press 2012). Since 2012, school-based vaccination rates have been rising in Ontario, but the 90 per cent target has never been reached (Graveland 2009; Puxley 2008; Stobbe 2011).

In the winter of 2010, Gardasil's indication was expanded to include boys and men up to twenty-six years of age (*CTVNews* 2010). In 2011, Health Canada also approved Gardasil for women up to forty-five years of age (Merck Frosst 2011a). After these regulatory approvals and expansions, NACI released an update in 2012 on the vaccine that supported vaccination for men up to twenty-six years of age and women up to forty-five years of age (see NACI 2012). In 2014, the Canadian

Immunization Committee (CIC) also advocated a gender-equity position with the recommendation to vaccinate both genders provincially, along with at-risk groups such as men who have sex with men (CIC 2014). In 2015, Health Canada approved Gardasil-9, which, as the name suggests, protects against nine strains of HPV (Merck Frosst 2015). The same year, NACI released another update on the vaccine, which focused on changing from a three-dose to a two-dose schedule for those who receive the vaccine when between the ages of nine and fourteen; all older or immunocompromised individuals, however, were advised to maintain the three-dose schedule (NACI 2015). This document is consistent with the 2012 NACI update in that it recommends the vaccine for boys, girls, men, and women (NACI 2015, 8). In 2017, NACI released a further update on the vaccine, which highlights recommendations to use either the HPV-2 in females and HPV-4 or HPV-9 vaccines in both males and females with a dose schedule as per the 2015 statement outlined above (NACI 2017). The report distinguishes between "good evidence" to support using HPV-2 and HPV-4 and "fair evidence" to use HPV-9 in healthy individuals (NACI 2017, 25). Thus, federal agencies have consistently advocated for gender parity when delivering the HPV vaccine in provincial programming or through private physician inoculation since 2012.

Accordingly, in April 2013, Prince Edward Island announced that it would fold boys into its existing grade 6 vaccination program, which had previously been geared towards girls only. Prince Edward Island positioned this policy development as a benevolent act towards women. Dr. Lamont Sweet, the deputy chief public health officer at the time, was quoted as saying, "boys can be the source of the virus for their female partners. By preventing boys from carrying the virus, you in turn will prevent girls from getting the virus which causes cervical cancer" (*CBC News* 2013). A few weeks later, the Government of Alberta announced that it too was looking into offering the vaccine to boys alongside grade 5 girls who were already being offered the shot. According to John Cotter (2013) of the Canadian Press, Alberta Health was to investigate the proposal in depth during the summer of 2013 and introduced the vaccine in 2014. Nova Scotia began offering the vaccine to boys in the fall of 2015, and the Government of British Columbia revealed that it would investigate inoculating "high-risk" boys, although the intended risk groups were not clear at the time of the announcement (*CBC News* 2015; Colbert 2015). Moreover, in the fall of 2016, the province of Ontario began vaccinating boys in their school-based programs (*CBC News* 2016), and in May 2017, Newfoundland announced that, starting in September of that year, boys would be inoculated in grade 6 along with the girls in their classes (Bartlett 2017). By 2019 the provincial HPV policy landscape had made some significant shifts, but this had been a long time coming. What accounts for this type of policymaking lag, particularly when provinces like Ontario, British Columbia, and Newfoundland only offered gender equity six or seven years after the vaccine was first approved by Health Canada for boys and men in 2010? The lobbying and marketing activity surrounding the vaccine as well as federal public policy concerning gender provide answers. I do, however, maintain throughout this book that despite these recent policy shifts, the HPV vaccine, and hence, HPV, is still branded as a women's issue in popular culture and the mind share of the general public in Canada. This is exhibited by the 2016 Society of Obstetricians and Gynaecologists of Canada (SOGC) advertisement campaign, outlined in chapter 5, which was geared toward women only.

Intensive Lobbying

It is not surprising that Merck Frosst, as a large pharmaceutical manufacturer, conducted lobbying activities in order to secure the regulatory approval of the HPV vaccine and its subsequent take-up in federal and provincial policymaking. Coverage of these activities focused on Ken Boessenkool, a former staff member of the Prime Minister's Office under Stephen Harper, who worked for the lobbying firm Hill+Knowlton and had acquired Merck Frosst as a client. Ken Boessenkool's connection to both Merck Frosst and the government of the day was heatedly discussed in the House of Commons (Government of Canada 2007) and numerous mainstream media outlets (Gillespie 2007; McGregor 2007; O'Malley 2007). Additionally, Merck Frosst's lobbying of the federal government can be traced through the lobby registry, which is run by the Office of the Commissioner of Lobbying of Canada. There are three listings for Merck Frosst on this registry that mention the HPV vaccine as a focus of its activities (see Office of the Commissioner of Lobbying of Canada 2007a, 2007b, 2008). In these entries, Merck Frosst discloses communications with the following federal departments: the Canadian International Development Agency; the Canadian International Trade Tribunal; the Federal Office of Regional Development – Quebec; Finance Canada, Foreign Affairs and International Trade Canada; Health Canada; Industry Canada; Justice Canada; Members of the House of Commons; National Research Council Canada; the Patented Medicine Prices Review Board; the Prime Minister's Office; the Privy Council Office; the Procurement Review Board of Canada; the Public Health Agency of Canada; Public Safety and Emergency Preparedness Canada;

the Senate of Canada; the Solicitor General of Canada; and the Treasury Board of Canada Secretariat. It is difficult to tease out, however, which departments were approached regarding the HPV vaccine specifically, as these contacts are listed as the result of the following policies or programs: Canada's Access to Medicines Regime; Health Canada's Blueprint for Renewal; Health Canada's Health Products and Foods Branch Cost Recovery Proposal for Human Drug User Fees; the Health Safety Action Plan; HPV Trust; the Patented Medicine Prices Review Board Pricing Guidelines; the Patented Medicine Prices Review Board Regulations; Patent Regulations; the Science and Technology Strategy; and the National Pharmaceutical Strategy (Office of the Commissioner of Lobbying of Canada 2008). This does indicate the limits of such disclosure mechanisms, as it is difficult to identify specific activities in its blanket format. Nevertheless, one can conclude that Merck Frosst was and is active in its lobbying activities to further its business objectives.

While pharmaceutical regulation is a federal responsibility in Canada, it is the provincial governments that carry out vaccine-related program planning and delivery. As such, there was also lobbying activity at the provincial level. In Ontario, for example, Tanya Talaga (2007) reported in the *Toronto Star* that Bob Lopinski, who had previously worked in Premier Dalton McGunity's office and who was working for Hill+Knowlton in 2007, and Jason Grier, who was previously the chief of staff to the former Health Minister George Smitherman and who also worked for Hill+Knowlton in 2007, lobbied the Ontario government on Merck Frosst's behalf in order to have the HPV vaccine rolled out in province-wide school-based programming. This information is also publicly available on the province of Ontario's lobbyist registry, which is hosted by the Office of the Integrity Commissioner.[1]

What is even more interesting, however, is Merck Frosst's indirect lobbying activities, which are extensive. As is covered in Wyndham-West, Wiktorowicz, and Tsasis (2017), Merck Frosst not only gave a $1.5-million grant to the SOGC for an informational campaign but also gave monies to other Canadian medical societies as well. As per Merck Frosst's public disclosure mechanism, the following medical societies listed in Table 2 were issued grants between 2007 and 2012.

Above and beyond the $1.5-million grant the SOGC received between 2007 and 2010, they accrued an additional $25,321 in 2011 and $290,000 in 2012. The collective monies granted to the four medical societies between 2007 and 2012 totalled $1,928,521. While the Merck Frosst disclosure documents do not detail the activities that resulted from these grants, all HPV vaccine activities the societies engaged in during the timeframe outlined above were publicly disclosed in the form of press

Table 2. Merck Frosst contributions to Canadian medical societies, 2007–12

Medical Society	Year(s)	Contribution ($)
Society of Obstetricians and Gynaecologists of Canada	2007–10	1,500,000
Federation of Medical Women of Canada	2009	1,000
Society of Gynecologic Oncology of Canada	2009	25,000
Federation of Medical Women of Canada	2010	7,500
Society of Gynecologic Oncology of Canada	2010	30,000
Society of Canadian Colposcopists	2011	7,500
Society of Gynecologic Oncology of Canada	2011	35,000
Society of Obstetricians and Gynaecologists of Canada	2011	25,321
Federation of Medical Women of Canada	2012	7,200
Society of Obstetricians and Gynaecologists of Canada	2012	290,000
Total		1,928,521

releases, policy position papers, and letters to the editors of various news-papers. For example, in 2006, the Society of Gynecologic Oncology of Canada (GOC) released a position statement backing the vaccine (GOC 2006). The Federation of Medical Women of Canada (FMWC) also sup-ported the vaccine through testimony at the Standing Committee on Finance in 2006. Dr. Gail Beck, then president of the FMWC, advocated for public, subsidized HPV vaccination campaigns to be available to both girls and boys. During her presentation to the federal Standing Commit-tee on Finance in Ottawa on the HPV vaccine, she argued, "I would cau-tion us to address this infection as one that is important to both men and women, thus the need to include both in any strategy. Clearly we need a national strategy that is informed by our diversity" (Standing Committee on Finance 2006). The FMWC's early attempts to "de-gender" (Paoletti 1997, 27) the vaccine were unique at this time.

In 2007, the Society of Canadian Colposcopists (SCC) and the GOC released position statements that supported the 2007 NACI statement on the approval and suggested programming attributes for the vaccine (GOC 2007; Society of Canadian Colposcopists 2007). Also in 2007, the College of Family Physicians of Canada released the *Canadian Con-sensus Guidelines on Human Papillomavirus*, which featured a link to the *Journal of Obstetrics and Gynaecology Canada* feature on the HPV vaccine (see SOGC 2007a). In 2012, the FMWC re-entered the public discourse surrounding the vaccine when its then president, Dr. Vivian Brown, was quoted by *the Canadian Press* as stating that "both sexes contribute to the transmission of HPV. Both sexes are at risk of developing a variety of HPV-related diseases – including cancer. So it follows that both sexes should be protected. But currently, that's not the case" (Branswell 2012). This advocacy had been ongoing and contributed to an expansion of the vaccine's indication to both genders when the NACI reworked its recommendation for the vaccine in 2012 to include both women and men (NACI 2012). At this time, the GOC again issued a statement in support of the NACI HPV vaccine guidelines (GOC 2012). In 2013, the CEO of the SOGC, Dr. Jennifer Blake, sent letters to provincial health ministers encouraging them to include boys (alongside the girls who were already being covered) in their school-based programs. This advocacy campaign was publicly announced in an SOGC press release on 25 April (*CMAJ* 2013).

Although the gender indication for the vaccine was officially expanded by the NACI in 2012, and despite the efforts of the FMWC and the SOGC to bring awareness to this angle of the vaccine at that time, the inclusion of boys was not folded into all provincial HPV vaccine delivery programs until the fall of 2017.

Gender-Based Analysis (GBA) Policy

Policy documents indicate that government officials at the federal level[2] examined the issue of the HPV vaccine within a GBA framework (Greaves 2009; Health Canada 2000, 2003a, 2003b; Standing Committee on the Status of Women 2005; Status of Women Canada 2004; Tudiver 2009). GBA is a policy development approach that the federal government has been using since the mid-1990s. The federal government first committed itself to using GBA in 1995 in conjunction with the Fourth World Conference on Women held in Beijing. That same year, the federal government released *The Federal Plan for Gender Equality*, a cornerstone document mapping its blueprint for GBA implementation (Status of Women Canada 1995). In 1999, Health Canada specifically committed itself to using GBA while developing policy and programs, and in 2003 it implemented a five-year plan to ensure that GBA would be in "full effect" across departmental initiatives (Health Canada 2003b). The goal of implementing GBA is to bring about gender equality in government programming and, hence, to the country as a whole (Hankivsky 2012a, 172). As the name indicates, GBA places a primacy on "gender as an essential variable in policy analysis" (Hankivsky 2012a, 172). Thus, gender is the pivotal axis through which policy is analysed and programs are developed, regardless of their aims or orientation. Health Canada (2003a, 1) describes GBA as a "catalyst for change," because GBA ensures that a "gender equality perspective" is folded into the development of health policy. Moreover, Health Canada (2003a, 1) uses GBA "to promote sound scientific research, and provide relevant health information and evidence." Accordingly, the framework has been adopted in women's health research conducted at Canadian universities and non-profit, health-oriented organizations (Abramson 2009; Jackson, Pederson, and Boscoe 2009; O'Sullivan and Amaratunga 2009). Such studies have examined topics as far reaching as communicable disease outbreaks and wait times for surgeries and diagnostic tests.

Within health research and program design, GBA is a tool that amplifies the difference between men and women and puts in place "a semblance of order," where difference on the ground is often difficult to demarcate (Douglas [1966] 2002, 5). Such a move works to "impose system on an inherently untidy experience" (Douglas [1966] 2002, 5). Therefore, conceptually, GBA in health research and program design pits men against women, views them as undifferentiated "wholes," and places a primacy on the effects of gender on health. Hankivsky (2012b) argues that much debate has taken place over the adoption and application of GBA in health research and program design, but not much discussion has been focused on the underlying theoretical tenets of the framework; she critiques GBA in health research and program design for its conceptual treatment of gender. In practice, the reference to gender within prevailing health-oriented GBA frameworks generally refers to women and not men. This pragmatic application of GBA is evident in the December 2007 CIC report on the HPV vaccine, which focused on cost-effectiveness analyses of the vaccine, a common policy exercise that is often an analytical subset of GBA. The cost-effectiveness model aims to develop policy that reaches the widest audience possible with "tangible" health benefits, all the while containing costs (Hankivsky 2007a). Vaccination programs tend to fare well in this type of analysis because the outcomes are simple to measure – the number of individuals vaccinated can easily be tallied.

The first cost-effectiveness analysis in the CIC (2007, 8) report focuses on females only, although the report does cite many studies in the bibliography on HPV that include both females and males. The authors chose not to bring this data into their analysis, thereby invoking gendering from the very beginning of the policymaking process. The second cost-effectiveness analysis in the CIC report includes boys, but no mention is made of potential HPV-related cancer rates in boys. In this analysis, the HPV vaccine is presented as an "altruistic" (Epstein 2010, 75) vaccine, and HPV as a "women's issue" – boys should be vaccinated to help eradicate cervical cancer in women. A third cost-effectiveness analysis can be found in a second document circulating around this same time, which was prepared for the Public Health Agency of Canada by the consulting firm H. Krueger and Associates. This report was not presented as a PHAC document but was nevertheless funded by the Agency. It also examines the cost-effectiveness of vaccinating girls and the eventual impact this will have on cervical cancer mortality rates. It concludes that there is no evidence to suggest that vaccinating boys will significantly reduce cervical cancer mortality (H. Krueger and Associates 2008, 32). Therefore, in these GBA modelling exercises, the ideal of "gender equality" translates into positioning women as needing much more assistance than their male counterparts, with women occupying a homogenous and static contingent of society, whose very essence – their gender – puts them at risk. In this sense, HPV vaccine–related policy processes have reinforced circulating gender norms, as many health policies do (Moore 2010, 100).

In addition to a lack of focus on both women and men, cost-effectiveness analyses do not invoke any form of "diversity analysis" (Hankivsky 2007b, 156) as it plays out within a gender grouping. For example, how does a woman's age, marital status, religion, geographic location, or income level affect her ability to take advantage of a specific program? As a case in point, women who do not have access to regular Pap screenings, such as many Indigenous, racialized, immigrant, homeless, or otherwise marginalized girls and women, are more susceptible to developing cervical cancer and make up a large portion of the approximately 400 cervical cancer deaths in Canada each year (CWHN 2007, 16). The issues these marginalized women face are not addressed in current HPV-related policy in Canada or Ontario. Thus, the concept of "female" that is plugged into HPV vaccine-oriented GBA frameworks insinuates that all women will encounter health-related challenges and barriers, regardless of class, race, age, or educational, religious, or geographical standing. GBA relies on the "assumption – either made implicitly or explicitly – that gender is the most frequent[ly] occurring, structural and important inequality for consideration" (Hankivsky 2012a, 174).

It is only fair to mention, though, that early GBA documentation did make reference to "diversity" among women. For example, *The Federal Plan for Gender Equality* states the following:

A gender-based approach ensures that the development, analysis and implementation of legislation and policies are undertaken with an appreciation of gender differences. This includes an understanding of the nature of relationships between men and women, and the different social realities, life expectations and economic circumstances facing women and men. It also acknowledges that some women may be disadvantaged even further because of their race, colour, sexual orientation, socio-economic position, region, ability level or age. A gender-based analysis respects and appreciates diversity. (Status of Women Canada 1995, 19)

This perspective, unfortunately, has not been applied in the case of the HPV vaccine.

HPV vaccine-oriented GBA offers a one-dimensional treatment of gender – or, more appropriately, women – which harkens back to standard second-wave feminist fare when scholars focused on the wide-sweeping subordination of women (Ortner 1974; Rosaldo 1974). While seeking to understand "why sexual asymmetry [is] a universal fact of human societies" (Rosaldo 1974, 22), academics developed totalizing theories to address this polemic. Michelle Rosaldo (1974, 41) posited that women's oppression stemmed from the positive cultural values associated with men's activities in the public sphere of business and politics, which were then contrasted with the negative cultural values associated with women's activities in the private sphere of the home. Sherry Ortner also drew on cultural associations of gender to account for the subjugation of women. Ortner (1974, 87) argued rather persuasively that women's inferior status was linked to their association with nature (mothering, breastfeeding, nurturing, and so on), whereas men were seen as belonging to culture (higher office, business, politics and general spheres of influence, and so on). Ortner's schema is particularly relevant to one of Merck Frosst's HPV vaccine advertising campaigns, which is directed at mothers. They are told in the advertisements that it is their specific duty to protect their daughters by getting them vaccinated (this campaign and mothers' reactions to it are covered in more detail in chapter 2). Rosaldo's and Ortner's theories still have saliency today, for these gendered cultural associations continue to circulate in medical, pharmaceutical, and governmental discourses. But their totalizing of women is problematic.

Not all women face subjection in the same way; one's class, age, education, geographic location, race, ethnicity, and religion also play a part, as has been explored more exhaustively in anthropology during the 1990s (see Abu-Lughod [1993] 2008; Di Leonardo 1998; Scheper-Hughes 1999; Tsing 1993; Visweswaran 1994) and in more recent feminist anthropology (see Bjork-James 2015; Bolles 2013; Craven and Davis 2013; Williams and Drew 2020). This scholarship, which coincides with third-wave feminism and post-feminism, focuses on the intersection of race, class, marginality, and gender around the globe. However, as Kamala Visweswaran states (1994, 75), "it is not enough to consider race, class, and sexuality as additive categories to a central concept" – the central concept being, of course, gender. All aspects of intersectionality need to be given due consideration. GBA's epistemological focus, which appears to be stuck in a previous analytical era, explains why Indigenous groups such as the Native Women's Association of Canada (NWAC) have been particularly displeased with GBA. In a 2007 report, the NWAC (2007, 6) declared, "Canada and others who have applied a GBA have failed to do so in a way that is sensitive to the multiple needs of Aboriginal women, who suffer not only from gendered discrimination, but racism and other forms of oppression. For example, Indigenous two-spirited women also suffer from discrimination based on their sexual orientation and women with disabilities also must deal with discrimination based on disability." The federal government's GBA approach to the HPV vaccine deploys a distilled and vexing conception of gender. While the federal government's motivations may be more benign than those of Merck Frosst – the government is not trying to sell vaccines – GBA is tasked with addressing a universal health disadvantage that women, as a homogenous group, will experience. Thus, all women are at risk all of the time.

Might we better serve women's health by taking a step back and reconceiving how the concept of gender is deployed in governmental policy and, as a result, how risk is attributed? Elizabeth Weed and Judith Butler urge just this. In reference to the invocation of GBA by international non-governmental bodies, such as United Nations agencies, Weed and Butler (2011) insist that

> gender is formed in relation to other social and political modes of social organization and is itself actively producing and reproducing such modes, including the family, labor, class, slavery, imperialism, immigration politics, and the state, to name a few ... Since gender is not an isolated factor or element on such a map, but is itself mobilized in a constitutive and productive relation to those other modes of organizing political life, the only way to gauge its usefulness is by tracking those effects. (4–5)

In this quotation, Weed and Butler attempt to establish gender as a wide-open concept, not one that is *entirely* predetermined. To further explain, one must acknowledge that gender "is a practice of improvisation within a scene of constraint ... [T]he terms that make up one's gender are, from the start, outside oneself in a sociality that has no single author (and that radically contests the notion of authorship itself)" (Butler 2004, 1). The constraint that Butler speaks about is demonstrated by the fact that policy – as well as pharmaceutical marketing campaigns – scripts subject formation.[3] Adriana Petryna (2002, 115–48) also notes that policy orders an individual's identity or sense of self and influences how this identity is communicated, interrogated, and absorbed into daily life. In the case of

HPV vaccine policy and pharmaceutical marketing strategies, the at-risk girl/woman comes into being. The at-risk girl/woman is firmly put in a box, as Douglas ([1966] 2002) described, in order to maintain societal order – in short, the gender asymmetrical status quo.

GBA+

In May 2013, the federal government announced it would be instituting an improved GBA framework called "GBA+." Status of Women Canada (2013) explained that "the 'plus' in the name highlights that gen-der-based analysis goes beyond gender, and includes the examination of a range of other intersecting identity factors (such as age, education, language, geography, culture and income)." Intersectionality (Crenshaw 1989) allows researchers to investigate the "simultaneous interactions between different aspects of social identity" (Hankivsky and Cormier 2009, 3), power structures, and health outcomes. Thus, factors such as gender and cultural patterns are examined within a holistic framework that also takes into account an individual's or collectivity's race/ethnicity, indigeneity, immigration/refugee patterns, class, sexuality, and religion. However, it is paramount to highlight that all of these social locations are mutually constituted and, additionally, socially constructed, elastic, and in constant production within a specific time and place (Weed and Butler 2011). One social location, such as gender or class, does not nec-essarily dominate as an influencer and predictor of health outcomes – all social locations intertwined will have an effect on health over the life course. As a result, intersectionality is not an "additive approach" (Hankivsky 2012b, 1713), whereby social locations are collected to assess their effect on health outcomes. Instead, the enmeshment of multiple social locations within power structures and hierarchies are analysed within their specific temporal context. Recent GBA+ literature explores the Canadian federal government's failure to meaningfully engage with GBA and GBA+ in matters of policymaking (Canadian Centre for Policy Alternatives 2019; Hankivsky and Mussell 2018), how GBA+ can be ap-plied to explicate Indigenous experiences and improve related policy outcomes (Findlay 2019; Flera and Maaka 2010), and how LGBTQ2+ perspectives can be integrated into state development and supported health policies (Mule 2020).

While it is too soon to evaluate the impact of the federal government's GBA+ initiative, Table 3, which outlines subsidized, school-based HPV vaccine programming across Canadian provinces as of the summer of 2017, calls for pause. As the table details, GBA has been extended to include boys, but gender is still the central, analytical axis. Visweswaran

Table 3. Subsidized HPV vaccine programs across Canada

Province	Age/Grade of School Vaccination Program	Girls	Boys	MSM or Vulnerable Groups	Catch-Up Programs	Number of Doses for School-Based Programs	4- or 9-Valent Vaccine	9-Valent Vaccine
Alberta	Grade 5	Yes	Yes, as of 2014	N/A	From 2014 to 2018, grade 9 boys were offered a catch-up program; all girls eligible until end of grade 12 (Alberta Health Services 2017)	3	9-valent	N/A
British Columbia	Grade 6, but can also be received through health care providers and public health units	Yes	Looking into "high risk" boys as of 2015 and decided to introduce Grade 6 vaccinations for boys in fall of 2017 (British Columbia Health 2017)	Free for females up to age twenty-six who are HIV+; MSM up to age twenty-six; boys in the care of Ministry of Children and Family Development; boys in youth custody centres (HealthLink BC 2017)	Free to all girls born between 1994 and 2004 who have not yet received the vaccine (HealthLink BC 2017)	2	9-valent	N/A
Manitoba	Grade 6 in schools for girls and grades 6, 8, or 9 for boys, but those eligible for subsidized vaccines can also access them for free at a doctor's office, public health office, nursing station, QuickCare Clinic, ACCESS Centre, or pharmacy	Yes	Yes, as of 2016 (Manitoba Health 2021)	N/A	"Once eligible always eligible" policy, so those who missed the vaccine at school can get it at a doctor's office, public health office, nursing station, QuickCare Clinic, ACCESS Centre, or pharmacy	2	4-valent	N/A

New Brunswick	Grade 7	Yes	Yes, as of 2017	N/A	Info could not be found	2, as of 2015 (MacKinnon 2017)	Info could not be found	N/A
Newfoundland and Labrador	Grade 6	Yes	Yes, as of 2017	Info could not be found	Info could not be found	Info could not be found	Info could not be found	N/A
Northwest Territories	No program	N/A	N/A	N/A	N/A	N/A	N/A	N/A
Nova Scotia	Grade 7	Yes	Yes, as of 2015	Info could not be found	Info could not be found	2 (Kraicer-Melamed and Quach 2017)	Info could not be found	N/A
Nunavut	No program	N/A	N/A	N/A	N/A	N/A	N/A	N/A
Ontario	Grade 8	Yes	Yes, as of September 2016	Free for MSM up to age twenty-six (Region of Waterloo n.d.)	Free of charge at local public health units for all under eighteen years of age (Government of Ontario 2017a)	2	4-valent	Not as of fall 2016
Prince Edward Island	Grade 6	Yes	Yes, as of 2013	Free for women up to age forty-five and men up to age twenty-six who have had unprotected sex with multiple partners, have a history of anal or genital warts, or missed the vaccine in grade 6; women who have had an abnormal Pap smear; anyone who is HIV+; MSM of any age (Fraser 2016)	Info could not be found	3	Info could not be found	N/A

(Continued)

Table 3. Subsidized HPV vaccine programs across Canada (*Continued*)

Province	Age/Grade of School Vaccination Program	Girls	Boys	MSM or Vulnerable Groups	Catch-Up Programs	Number of Doses for School-Based Programs	4- or 9-Valent Vaccine	9-Valent Vaccine
Quebec	Grade 4	Yes	Yes, as of 2016 (Government of Quebec n.d.)	Free for MSM up to age twenty-six and for those who are immunocompromised or HIV+	Catch-up programs for girls up to seventeen years of age	2	9-valent	Yes, as of 2016
Saskatchewan	Grade 6	Yes	Yes, as of 2017	N/A	Girls born since 1997 can get the vaccine free at local health centres until they are twenty-seven years of age (Government of Saskatchewan 2017)	N/A	4-valent	N/A
Yukon	No program	N/A	N/A	N/A	N/A	N/A	N/A	N/A

Note: Data sourced 15 August 2017.

(1994) warned against keeping gender as the primary axis of analysis while adding on other positionality factors for consideration. However, this prediction does not bear out below as intersectional factors are not brought into consideration. For example, how are marginalized or Indigenous women incorporated into policymaking? The province of Ontario did extend the shot free of charge to all men who have sex with men (MSM) up to the age of twenty-six in 2016 (Canadian Press 2016a), but why have the other provinces not followed suit? How about individuals who are HIV+ and particularly susceptible to developing HPV-related cancers? More policy work needs to be focused in this area, and intersectionality needs to be meaningfully integrated into GBA. However, before offering policy solutions going forward, we will take a step back and examine why gender remains the dominant analytical lens in public health policymaking regarding the HPV vaccine.

Conclusion

This chapter highlights the vast network of stakeholders Merck Frosst leveraged through direct and indirect lobbying while introducing the HPV vaccine to Canada to ensure its successful take-up in federal and provincial policymaking. It is crucial to highlight that during the initial period of federal and Ontario provincial endorsements of the vaccine for use in girls and women, scientific literature on HPV, particularly epidemiological studies, was gender blind. This literature generally focused on the linkage between HPV and male, female, and multi-gendered cancers (see Munoz et al. 2006; Parkin and Bray 2006). In 2008, Dr. Harald zur Hausen, the Nobel Prize winner who discovered the link between HPV and cervical cancer, publicly questioned (and continues to question) the gendering of HPV-related vaccines and suggested that boys also should have been inoculated from the start, as is public health policy in Austria (Zechmeister, Freiesleben de Blasio, and Garnett 2010). The point here is that science/medicine did not gender HPV and the vaccine. This was a governmental rendering; federal and provincial governments devised and carried out gendered policies, which were based on Merck Frosst's marketing lead, which was described in chapter 5. Importantly, though, Merck Frosst would not have been able to gender a virus, and hence their vaccine, no matter how much money they spent on direct or indirect lobbying, if hegemonic cultural notions of women did not support and reinforce the notion that girls and women are perpetually at risk and need assistance to mitigate this risk.

7 Conclusion: Theoretical Contributions and Reassessing Gender-Based Analysis Policymaking

Research and Analysis Summary

This book has been an endeavour in answering three overarching questions: (1) How did the HPV vaccine become gendered within the Canadian policy landscape, and how did this in turn lead to gendered public health programming? (2) How do women appropriate, hybridize, or refute the notions of "gender" and "risk" that are deployed in association with the vaccine? and (3) How were their experiences with risk and gender folded into their vaccine decision-making? To answer these questions, fieldwork took on two phases. In the first phase, the creation and circulation of the concepts of "gender" and "risk" that were deployed in pharmaceutical and policy discourses vis-à-vis the HPV vaccine were tracked through archival research comprising Gardasil advertising campaigns, national media coverage, parliamentary debates, federal and provincial press releases, accounts of lobbying before the federal finance committee, and federal regulatory decisions regarding the vaccine. As policy documents indicate, the federal government developed HPV vaccine policy within a GBA framework, which followed the parameters of Merck Frosst's gender-based marketing. Such gender "ideals" rest upon the overarching notion that women are a "feminine" grouping – a homogenous and static "whole" that is inherently at risk for ill health. Merck Frosst was the first to deploy these governance techniques as a selling mechanism for the vaccine and was very skilled at deploying these across multiple platforms in direct and indirect lobbying activities. If these conceptualizations were not already out there in the ether, they would not have been picked up again in policymaking. Within the policy sphere, like in other realms of daily life, static, cultural "ideals" of gender and risk circulate widely.

The archival contextualization provided the requisite background to conduct the second phase of research, the tracing of how the concepts of risk and gender were mediated by two different groups of women: mothers negotiating the vaccine for their daughters in a school-based immunization program and university students who were targets of HPV vaccine promotion in campus health clinics. It was not particularly surprising to discover that a multinational pharmaceutical company led governmental policy development, although chapters 4, 5 and 6 do detail the intricate, multi-pronged strategies deployed by pharmaceutical companies through direct and indirect lobbying, including message deployment and reverberation throughout the national media. The governance net that is woven by corporate interests is both vast and tight. This book brings into relief how women negotiate conceptualizations of risk and gender that are informed by private interests within everyday contexts. I sought to understand how women folded these concepts into their vaccine decision-making. Perhaps risk was emphasized more than gender, or was it the other way around? In answering these questions, the vicissitudes of power – as it was deployed and how it was processed – were examined.

In order to analyse the data gathered, Foucault's early and late theory ([1969] 1989, [1978] 1990, 1987, 1991, 1997, 1999) was utilized. Additionally, Douglas's ([1966] 2002, 1992) work on risk and the work of those who follow the governmentality school of risk (Castel 1991; C. Gordon 1991; Lupton 1994, 1995, 1999a, 1999b, 2003; Lupton and Petersen 1996; Nettleton 1997; Petersen 1997; Rose 2007; Rothstein 2006; Turner 1997) was brought into the theoretical fold. Governmentality approaches have been critiqued for their predetermined nature (Sawicki 1991, 98), but once I examined the continuum of this work, tightly woven governance strategies began to loosen and, one could even say, unravel. By examining Foucault's work on its continuum, I was able to acknowledge the construction of subjects within the framework of power relations as well as the possibility that such subjects could level their own "critique" while enmeshed in power networks (Allen 2008, 21). Women's narratives provided an intersubjective space wherein subject formation and realizations/actualizations of the self intersected, and it was in this space that health negotiation and decision-making occurred. In this intersubjective space, women worked towards becoming "ethical" beings by creating their own "telos" or sets of codes for manoeuvring daily life (Foucault 1997, 265). Scripting one's telos is a limited act of power and is reflected in women's ability to be "self-constituting" (Allen 2008, 2).

The use of early and late Foucault theory, along with writings by Allen (2008), Butler (2008), Nettleton (1997), Lupton (1999b), and Zaloom

(2004), allowed for the analysis of situated risk (Boholm 2003) *and* gender. This is where this book makes its greatest contribution to existing social science literature related to risk, which generally zeroes in on either grand theory (see Beck 2004; Castel 1991; Dean 1999; Ewald 1991; N. Fox 1997; Giddens 1991; C. Gordon 1991; Petersen 1997; Rothstein 2006) *or* individual accounts (see Bond et al. 2012; Brown et al. 2013; Crighton et al. 2013; Gross and Shuval 2008; Lear 1995; Russell and Kelly 2011; Spencer 2013; Thing and Ottesen 2013; Tuinstra et al. 1998; Walls et al. 2010; Zinn 2008). Concentrating solely on grand theory leaves out the important human element of risk, and exclusively researching individual experiences unintentionally reproduces sales/governance strategies. However, as important as research focusing on situated risk is, it is usually not extended to issues relating to gender in a critical fashion (Lupton 1999a). Moore (2010) also notes that if gender is addressed in situated risk research, it is treated with such limited theorization that findings usually reinforce gender norms. This book addresses this void in the academic record by treating both the concepts of risk and gender with critical care, all the while producing ethnographic accounts of women's experiences negotiating risk *and* gender.

Theoretical Contributions

Ontological Decision-Making Framework

Numerous ethnographic examples of women taking a pause and crafting their narratives of self and identity populate the medical anthropology/sociology literature (see Becker 1999; Garro 2000; Gregg 2003, 2011; Hunt 2000; Kirmayer 2000; Kohler Riessman 2000; Pandolfi 2007; Rapp 2007; Saukko 2010; Thompson 2005, 2007; Throsby 2010). However, something quite specific took place when women spoke of their decisions around whether or not to have their daughters or themselves vaccinated against HPV. In an overarching sense, their ethical agency involved aspects of Thompson's (2005) "ontological choreography," which entails the "dynamic coordination" of various aspects of self. In the case of some students, ontological choreography was fleetingly accompanied by the "biographical disruption" (Bury 1982) of being ill in the form of persistent cervical dysplasia. However, women's ethical agency in the pause also pointedly involved the reordering of gender and risk across both cohorts. For the women interviewed, risk and gender intersected in a "productive" (Zaloom 2004) manner. In other words, risk and gender were practised when vaccine decision-making occurred. HPV vaccine decision-making provided the key to the door to understanding how gender and risk were appropriated to varying degrees of importance (to answer research question two), and when health decisions were made (to answer research question three). These decisions were linked to the women's senses of self, with conceptualizations of risk and gender differing depending on where a woman was in her life cycle.

When ontological choreography and biological disruption intersected, women consciously engaged in reordering. Thus, the concepts of risk and gender were movable ontological modes; risk and gender shifted in and out of focus depending on the context, but they were always present in some form, no matter how subtle. For mothers, risk was a theoretical construct; their daughters were just moving into their teenage years, and so they tended to view HPV risk as a distant proposition. Mothers thus focused on gender and doing mothering. For students, many of whom had experienced transient HPV infections in the form of genital warts and low-grade cervical dysplasia, focus was on HPV risk and potential vaccine side effects. They were also angry with the gendering of HPV and the vaccine and based their vaccination decisions on the type of gendered being they would like to be – one not put in a predetermined box of being at risk. Students were, therefore, dealing both with risk and gender simultaneously. Thus, in response to the creation and circulation of the gendered and risky HPV-related subject formations – which attempt to keep women "in order" and prompt them to "follow orders" – women reordered *their* lives.

Reordering presents both a threat to order and the potential to enact power (Douglas [1966] 2002, 117). Thus, while doing, women are creatively reappropriating/rejecting and hybridizing the gendered and risky HPV subject formation to productive effect. Butler (2008) describes this process of reordering within the parameters of existing norms:

> There is no making of oneself (*poiesis*) outside of a mode of subjectivation (*assujettissement*) and, hence, no self-making outside of the norms that orchestrate the possible forms that a subject may take. The practice of critique will thus expose the limits of the historical scheme of things, the epistemological and ontological horizon within which subjects come to be at all. To make oneself, then, in such a way that one exposes those limits is precisely to engage an aesthetics of the self that maintains a critical relation to existing norms. (26–7)

Correspondingly, it was ironic how mothers played with the concept of the good mother and students rejected mainstream concepts of gender and risk when saying "no" to the vaccine, a rejection germane to their generation's conceptualizations of gender and emerging womanhood.

Figure 2. Reordering of risk and gender

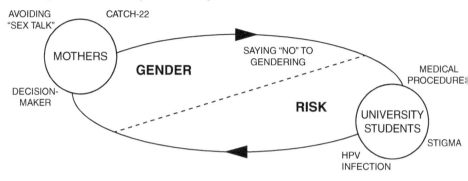

Nevertheless, while working within existing norms, each woman did this on her own terms. Risk and gender were folded into the women's senses of self in myriad ways shared across, between, and within each cohort.[1] What governance strategies had tried to "fix," the women interviewed continually unfixed and re-fixed, each in her own way. This process, or reordering, then, undermines the dominant order and provides the potential to enact power. This process is represented in Figure 2.

Women's accounts of situated risk and gender also indicated that they were engaged in ontological decision-making around whether or not to get vaccinated or to have their daughters vaccinated. As women reordered, they were also "doing." Mothers were doing mothering and students were doing gender politics and experiencing intermittent risk. In carrying out each aspect of "doing," women wove nets or nests of experiences, which, when assembled, helped form their ethical being or sense of self. The knowledge accumulated through situated risk and gender experiences was then layered to inform vaccination decisions. Figure 3 outlines the circular and nest-like processes of ontological decision-making. As an inherently social and cultural process, ontological decision-making is embedded in women's experiences of finding meaning in their efforts to be good mothers and strong young women made to feel vulnerable in sexual health negotiation.

In developing the concept of ontological decision-making, I aim to demonstrate how women made vaccine decisions based on their risk and gender-related negotiation experiences and not in terms of a linear, cost-benefit analysis. In this way, this book departs from existing literature on risk-related decision-making. Research on decision-making posits it as the result of linear, cost-benefit analyses (Austin et al. 2013; Jacobson, Targonski, and Poland 2007; Poland and Jacobson 2001; Poland, Jacobson, and Ovsyannikova 2009). For example, Crighton et al.

Figure 3. Nested decisions to form the frameworks of ontological decision-making

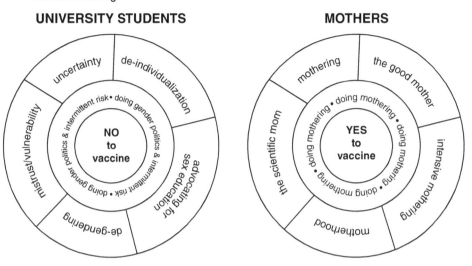

UNIVERSITY STUDENTS   MOTHERS

(2013, 298) argue that such approaches involve "two cognitive mediating processes: the threat appraisal process [that] evaluates the potential benefits of action as well as the availability of resources (financial or other) to do so." This type of linear, cost-benefit analysis also positions decision-making as a "rational" and individual act. Thus, when individuals do not follow risk prevention directives, they are often cast as ill-informed or as not being able to grasp the complexity of the risk issue at hand (Lupton 1999a, 2). This approach does not recognize that decision-making is "more a process than an isolated action" (Hobson-West 2010, 280). In short, it misses the "situatedness" of risk (and gender for that matter). Ontological decision-making is an inherently social and cultural process, which is embedded in women's experiences of "mobilizing meanings" (McClure 1992, 365) surrounding their efforts to be good mothers and strong young women merging into adulthood amidst the anxiety of intermittent HPV infection risk and the worry about potential risks the vaccine may or may not bring.

Sales/Governance Strategies

This book, through the case study of the HPV vaccine, highlights how corporations and governments work hand in hand to set public health policy in the neo-liberal era of the new public health. Merck Frosst, the

Government of Canada, and many provincial governments deployed vaccine marketing, information, mainstream media coverage, and public health programming to influence women to get vaccinated through self-regulation. This individualized approach facilitated the sale of the vaccine and reinforced the governance tenets of the new public health, which emphasizes a self-disciplining approach to regulating populations. Both Merck Frosst and the Canadian and provincial governments framed HPV as a "women's issue" by cleverly harnessing existing hegemonic cultural ideals surrounding risk and gender already in circulation. The gendering of HPV aided in creating a "need" for the vaccine and the related in-school vaccination programming.

Generative Pause

In researching situated risk and gender, it became clear that when women spoke about their experiences navigating risk, gender, and the vaccine, the pause they took during interviews was indeed a generative moment. Not only were interviews times of contemplation, but they were also productive events. Mothers and students ruminated and processed how HPV infection and HPV vaccine risk was being transmitted through governmental and pharmaceutical discourses and how they themselves were hybridizing or rejecting these messages. However, women were communicating much more than their vaccine decision-making processes during interviews. When taking a pause, each woman created a narrative that contributed to her continually developing sense of self. As each narrative developed, identity was reinscribed and re-enforced, for it was in the thick of the pause that the exterior subject formation imposed by pharmaceutical and governmental discourses and interior realizations/actualizations of the self intersected. Women are not always portrayed as "doers," and in the case of HPV infection and the vaccine women are positioned as passive recipients and bearers of disease. It was in the space of the pause that women actively, continually, and complexly negotiated their senses of self while working to secure their health vis-à-vis HPV infection and the HPV vaccine.

The Productive Reordering of Risk and Gender

It is important to note that women were not reinforcing the gendered at-risk subject formation of pharmaceutical and governmental discourses when they were doing mothering, doing gender politics, and experiencing intermittent risk. Sales/governance strategies attempt to order individuals or groups. In response, women reordered *their* lives. Reordering presents both a threat to established orders of power and the potential to enact power. Thus, while "doing," women were creatively reappropriating/rejecting and hybridizing the gendered and risky HPV subject formation to productive effect. As a result, the women of each cohort were doing their making of self differently, depending on their context. It was ironic how mothers played with the concept of the good mother and students rejected mainstream concepts of gender and risk when saying "no" to the vaccine. Each woman was doing this in her own way. Women did not exhibit one universal formula for interpreting gender and risk that mirrored the flat and totalizing way in which gendered risk is constructed and deployed in pharmaceutical and governmental policy discourses vis-à-vis the HPV vaccine.

Either combined or used independently, the four concepts of sales/governance strategies, the generative pause, the productive reordering of risk and gender, and ontological decision-making provide novel frames through which to engage in and analyse situated risk and gender research.

Pragmatic Policy Considerations Going Forward

The lessons learned from the roll-out of the HPV vaccine in Ontario, and within Canada more broadly, suggest two potential policy measures: (1) direct and indirect lobbying activities of pharmaceutical companies should be registered in Canada so that their sales/governance strategies and activities are transparent to the public; and (2) gender-based analysis policy frameworks need to be reworked to take into account disease specificity and the fluidity of gender constructs. These proposed policy measures are explained more fully here:

1 *Registering direct and indirect pharmaceutical lobbying.* As chapters 4, 5, and 6 demonstrate, the tentacles of pharmaceutical sales/governance strategies have a wide and deep reach. Tracing these direct and indirect strategies is a time-consuming and laborious task – one that is far too onerous to expect of individuals trying to decide which vaccines and medicines to take. In the spirit of informed health decision-making consent, federal legislation that parallels Ontario's proposed Health Sector Payment Transparency Act (2017) is required (see Government of Ontario 2017b). Under this legislation, pharmaceutical companies would have to disclose the payments they make to patient-advocacy groups and professional medical societies. This is intended to provide transparency to the monies funnelled from pharmaceutical companies to health charities and non-profit

organizations. The data unearthed in chapter 6, which outlines how much Merck Frosst paid to medical societies between 2007 and 2012, should be information that is easily accessible to the public through a central information source, as is outlined in the proposed Health Sector Payment Transparency Act. Under this act, failure to report payments could result in fines of up to $100,000 a day for non-compliance (Grant 2018). The proposed legislation also extends beyond patient-advocacy groups and medical societies to health researchers and clinicians and would require "pharmaceutical companies and medical device makers to disclose all financial interactions with clinicians, health practitioners, researchers and educators" (Brown 2018). Under this act it would be "up to the payer to communicate information to the Ministry, who will collect, analyse, publish and audit this information on a public website" (Brown 2018). The legislation was expected come into effect in 2018 with a searchable database available for viewing in 2020, however, with the election of a Conservative provincial government in June of 2018, this legislation was put on pause (Owens 2019). Ontario has thus far been the only Canadian province to consider such legislation, and the other provinces and the federal government should follow suit.

2 *Transforming GBA frameworks within health policy development to take into account disease specificity, the fluidity of gender constructs, and underserviced groups.* The best way to describe how GBA frameworks, particularly GBA+ frameworks, should work in public health policy is to describe what the optimal policy and programming for HPV vaccine access should look like. Ideally, a GBA+ framework would have captured the following components when putting together policy and programming frameworks. First, the vaccine should have been considered for all genders from the outset. This would have required, however, a solid grasp of HPV infection etiology, which is gender blind. As such, policymakers should receive medical/scientific briefs in easy-to-understand language explaining how the specific virus/illness/disease is transferred. Without this basic scientific information, policymakers are making decisions with only one eye open. Second, gender should be conceptualized in nuanced ways, as not all women or all men, depending upon their social location, are at risk for specific diseases and illnesses. In the case of HPV, underserviced and marginalized women are most at risk of succumbing to cervical cancer, so where is the policy and programming to address these women?

Unfortunately, the introduction of GBA+ in 2013 has not borne out equitable HPV vaccine policy and programming frameworks in Ontario or across Canada. This book is an attempt at bringing this into focus. GBA+ needs to be implemented in a more nuanced way with a full understanding of the fluid and moving relationships between gender and intersectionality as suggested by Hankivsky and Cormier (2009). In order to do so, policymakers should be asked the following questions:

- Where are the programs for Indigenous or homeless women in Ontario and across Canada who are far more likely to die of cervical cancer than women who have access to regular Pap tests?
- Have MSM received free HPV vaccination in Ontario due to successful activism while vulnerable women have not because they do not have access to similar activism?
- Should the onus be on advocacy groups, such as MSM activists in Ontario, to drive health policy and programming, or should the government be driving equitable policymaking?

I argue that GBA+ policymaking processes should be immune to the reach and influence of stakeholders, whether that be public health groups, medical societies, or pharmaceutical manufacturers. As this book has demonstrated, their reach in matters of policymaking in Canada is wide and their grip tight. This should cause us all pause and provide the springboard to develop and implement meaningful policymaking frameworks going forward to ensure optimal health for all individuals, regardless of their ability to access resources to advocate for health policy change.

Notes

1. Introduction

1 This use of risk is not meant to propagate Ulrich Beck's (2000, 216) notion of "manufactured uncertainty." Manufactured uncertainty refers to risk that is a product of and a factor inherent to modernity. While Beck (2000, 212) argues that he is both a realist and a constructivist, his writings veer more to the realist side of the risk equation than governmentality approaches to risk, which emphasize the construction of risk as a governance technique.

2 Although, Boholm (2003) does not refer to Lock and Kaufert (1998) in her piece, situated risk and situated gender are issue-specific versions of producing "situated accounts" of the "microphysics of power" (Lock and Kaufert 1998, 1) as they play out in the everyday realm of HPV vaccine negotiation and decision-making.

3 Lupton also fuses governmentality and cultural approaches to risk in her research.

4 Foucault's exclusive use of masculine pronouns is problematic in both this quote and his work overall. Theory has also been drawn from Allen (2008), Butler (2008), Douglas ([1966] 2002, 1992), Lupton (1999a, 1999b), Moore (2010), and Nettleton (1996, 1997) in order to incorporate a feminist lens into the analysis.

5 The approach taken throughout my fieldwork was also political, underscored by the theoretical underpinnings of the research project.

6 As an example of such an approach and results, Scott discusses E.P. Thompson's work. In looking to contest the closed nature of the category of "class," Thompson positioned experience as a state of "social being – the lived realities of social life" (quoted in Scott 1992, 29). While this take on experience does allow for agentive aspects of experience to emerge, Thompson's analysis rests firmly

upon the affects/effects of the "relations of production," thereby reaffirming class as a "unifying phenomenon, overriding other kinds of diversity" (Scott 1992, 29).

7 Dana Lear (1995, 1317) also found that young adults reported that the sex education they received before university was "woefully inadequate."

2. Navigating Controversies and Doing Mothering: Making HPV Vaccine Decisions for One's Daughter

1 At the time, the vaccine was approved by Health Canada only for women and girls from nine to twenty-six years of age.

2 This is a high educational attainment rate when compared to Canada overall. In 2007, just under 25 per cent of Canadians held a university degree (Conference Board of Canada n.d.).

3 I did not, however, have the opportunity to interview lesbian mothers. I did send out a call for interviewees to various organizations where this participation would seem more likely, but I received no responses.

4 Biehl, Good, and Kleinman (2007, 7, 10) also make reference to the term "intersubjective." In their volume the term denotes experiences across or among a grouping of individuals or collectivities.

5 Please note that this document is not formally cited, as to do so would reveal the residential location of many interviewees.

6 See the published reports of Cancer Care Ontario for statistics and trends: https://www.cancercareontario.ca/en/statistical-reports/ontario-cancer -statistics-2020/ch-6cancer-mortality-rates-trends.

7 I approached Merck Frosst for copyright permission to reproduce its advertisements in this book. After several months, Merck Frosst responded by email to say that permission could be obtained if I signed a legal agreement that the text accompanying the images in my book would not reflect negatively upon Merck Frosst and that Merck Frosst would be the arbiter of what is considered negative. I, of course, did not sign the agreement. Even though academic critique of Merck Frosst advertisements could be considered "fair dealing" under Canadian copyright law, Merck Frosst promotional materials have not been used in this book.

8 This framing is similar to the contact between what Foucault describes as subject formation and the development of one's sense of self or ethics (Allen 2008), as discussed earlier in this chapter.

9 Being a mother is but one identity ascription of the women interviewed. Women also identified as professional working individuals, sisters, aunts, partners, daughters, and so forth, but during interviews their focus was on mothering strategies.

3. University-Aged Women's Experiences with HPV Infection and Vaccine Decision-Making

1 A low-risk HPV strain, as opposed to a high-risk HPV strain, is not oncogenic, meaning cancer causing. Strains of HPV that cause genital warts are not thought to turn into cancer (National Cancer Institute 2012).
2 While one might assume that Sylvana got the HPV infection from her boyfriend, this may not necessarily have been the case. She may have been the carrier without initial symptoms and the one to transfer it to her boyfriend. HPV is a complex virus, and infection pathways are not always linear. This often adds to public misunderstandings of HPV.
3 Virginity as defined as having had no vaginal intercourse does not necessarily preclude contracting HPV. Any form of genital touching can expose someone to HPV (Gilman, Gilman, and Johns 2009).
4 Gardasil was granted approval for use by boys and men up to the age of twenty-six by Health Canada in February 2010 (*CTVNews* 2010).
5 Amber's blog post has been paraphrased here as the original post can still be found on the Web and could be used to identify her.
6 While different publications list different numbers, HPV is generally reported as having over 100 different strains (Society of Obstetricians and Gynaecologists of Canada 2012).
7 Whether or not this form of "negative agency" (Wardlow 2006) puts students at risk should be debated, but this is not the focus of the research. Public health policymakers and communicators should take note of how gendered framing affects vaccine decision-making outcomes.
8 It is important to note that students did not speak about being targeted because of their age. Discourses surrounding youth and risk are rife in public health programming (see Brown et al. 2013; Spencer 2013; Thing and Ottesen 2013) and society in general (Giroux 2010), but students ranged in age from twenty to twenty-eight, and they did not consider themselves to be "youth."
9 Although students wished for the state to re-engage with sexual health education, they were not engaging in Beck's notion of subpolitics when opting out of being vaccine consumers. As such, students were not taking part in the "re-politicization of areas outside the iron cage of bureaucratic politics" (Holzer and Sørensen 2003, 80), but were seeking to reinsert themselves into governmental apparatuses.

6. Gendered Vaccine Policymaking

1 For Ontario's lobbyist registry, see https://lobbyist.oico.on.ca/Pages /Public/PublicSearch.

2 While public health issues are theoretically under provincial jurisdiction in Canada, the drive to bring the HPV vaccine to Canada occurred at the federal level. Not only is the federal government charged with approving pharmaceutical products, but it was also responsible for allocating the initial $300 million for transfer to the provinces on a per capita basis to get the vaccination programs started.

3 Giroux (2010, 7–8) argues that neo-liberalism is "also a political project, intent on producing new forms of subjectivity and sanctioning particular modes of conduct." Merck Frosst's campaign brings this point into relief.

7. Conclusion: Theoretical Contributions and Reassessing Gender-Based Analysis Policymaking

1 Rayna Rapp (1994) also found great variety within and across class groupings when she interviewed New York City women regarding amniocentesis. In my study, class is not used as a marker because most women interviewed were middle class.

References

Abramson, Beth. 2009. "Women and Health: Taking the Matter to Heart."
    In *Women's Health: Intersections of Policy, Research and Practice*, edited by Pat
    Armstrong and Jennifer Deadman, 53–60. Toronto: Women's Press.
Abu-Lughod, Lila. (1993) 2008. *Writing Women's Worlds: Bedouin Stories.* Los
    Angeles: University of California Press. https://doi.org/10.1525
    /9780520934979.
Alberta Health Services. 2017. "Human Papillomavirus 9-Valent Vaccine Biological
    Page." Last modified 1 January 2021. http://www.albertahealthservices.ca
    /assets/info/hp/cdc/If-hp-cdc-hpv-bio-pg-07-241.pdf.
Allen, Amy. 2008. *The Politics of Our Selves: Power, Autonomy, and Gender in
    Contemporary Critical Theory.* New York: Columbia University Press. https://
    doi.org/10.7312/alle13622.
Appadurai, Arjun. 1990. "Disjuncture and Difference in the Global Cultural
    Economy." *Theory, Culture & Society* 7, no. 2–3 (June): 295–310. https://doi
    .org/10.1177/026327690007002017.
Associated Press. 2008. "HPV Vaccine Prevents Genital Warts in Males." *Waterloo
    Region Record*, 14 November 2008.
Austin, Laurel C., Susanne Reventlow, Peter Sandoe, and John Brodersen.
    2013. "The Structure of Medical Decisions: Uncertainty, Probability and Risk
    in Five Common Choice Situations." *Health, Risk & Society* 15 (1): 27–50.
    https://doi.org/10.1080/13698575.2012.746286.
Bartky, Sandra. 1990. *Femininity and Domination: Studies in the Phenomenology of
    Oppression.* New York: Routledge. https://doi.org/10.4324/9780203825259.
Bartlett, Geoff. 2017. "Offering HPV Vaccine to Boys Finally Ends 'Sexist'
    Policy, Says Tonsil Cancer Survivor." *CBC News*, 5 May 2017. https://www.cbc
    .ca/news/canada/newfoundland-labrador/hpv-vaccine-boys-newfoundland
    -glenn-deir-1.4100762.
Beauvoir, Simone de. 1952. *The Second Sex.* Translated by H.M. Parshley. New
    York: Knopf.

Beck, Ulrich. 2000. "Risk Society Revisited: Theory, Politics and Research Programmes." In *The Risk Society and Beyond: Critical Issues for Social Theory*, edited by Barbara Adam, Ulrich Beck, and Joost Van Loon, 211–29. London: Sage Publications. https://doi.org/10.4135/9781446219539.

Beck, Ulrich, and Johannes Willms. 2004. *Conversations with Ulrich Beck*. Translated by Michael Pollack. Cambridge: Polity Press.

Becker, Gay. 1999. *Disrupted Lives: How People Create Meaning in a Chaotic World*. Berkeley: University of California Press.

Beilin, Caren. 2021. "Medicine and Misogyny." *Art in America*, 8 October 2021. https://www.artnews.com/art-in-america/interviews/feminist-health-care-research-group-caren-beilin-1234606473.

Berman, Hershel. 2008. "Unjust HPV Rule." Letter to the editor, *Globe and Mail*, 5 June 2008. https://www.theglobeandmail.com/opinion/letters/unjust-hpv-rule/article959617.

Biehl, João. 2007. "Pharmaceutical Governance." In *Global Pharmaceuticals: Ethics, Markets, Practices*, edited by Adriana Petryna, Andrew Lakoff, and Arthur Kleinman, 206–39. Durham, NC: Duke University Press. https://doi.org/10.1215/9780822387916-008.

Biehl, João, Byron Good, and Arthur Kleinman. 2007. "Introduction: Rethinking Subjectivity." In *Subjectivity: Ethnographic Investigations*, edited by João Biehl, Byron Good, and Arthur Kleinman, 1–23. Berkeley: University of California Press. https://doi.org/10.1525/california/9780520247925.003.0001.

Bjork-James, Sophie. 2015. "Feminist Ethnography in Cyberspace: Imagining Families in the Cloud." *Sex Roles* 73, no. 3–4 (June): 113–24. https://doi.org/10.1007/s11199-015-0507-8.

Blackwell, Tom. 2007. "For One Mother, There Is No Doubt; Controversial Cancer Vaccine Stirs Difficult Debate." *National Post*, 24 September 2007.

– 2008. "Vaccine Could End Most Cervical Cancer: Study; HPV Shots Urged for Older Women." *National Post*, 21 April 2008, A1.

– 2016a. "Journal Permanently Spikes Canadian Co-authored Study of HPV Vaccine." *National Post*, 8 March 2016. https://nationalpost.com/news/canada/journal-permanently-spikes-canadian-study-critical-of-hpv-vaccine.

– 2016b. "Medical Journal Yanks Study That Questions Safety of HPV Vaccine." *National Post*, 18 February 2016. https://nationalpost.com/health/medical-journal-yanks-study-that-questions-safety-of-hpv-vaccine.

Blatchford, Andy. 2011. "Researchers Pay More Attention to HPV as a Source of Mouth, Throat Cancers." *Toronto Star*, 10 May 2011. https://www.thestar.com/life/health_wellness/diseases_cures/2011/05/10/researchers_pay_more_attention_to_hpv_as_a_source_of_mouth_throat_cancers.html.

Blume, Stuart. 2006. "Anti-vaccination Movements and Their Interpretations." *Social Science & Medicine* 62, no. 3 (February): 628–42. https://doi.org/10.1016/j.socscimed.2005.06.020.

Boholm, Asa. 2003. "Situated Risk: An Introduction." *Ethnos* 68 (2): 157–8. https://doi.org/10.1080/0014184032000097713.

Bolles, Lynn. 2013. "Telling the Story Straight: Black Feminist Intellectual Thought in Anthropology." *Transforming Anthropology* 21, no. 1 (March): 57–71. https://doi.org/10.1111/traa.12000.

Bond, Chelsea, Mark Brough, Geoffrey Spurling, and Noel Hayman. 2012. "'It Had to Be My Choice': Indigenous Smoking Cessation and Negotiations of Risk, Resistance and Resilience." *Health, Risk & Society* 14 (6): 565–81. https://doi.org/10.1080/13698575.2012.701274.

Bourdieu, Pierre. 1977. *Outline of a Theory of Practice.* Cambridge: Cambridge University Press. https://doi.org/10.1017/CBO9780511812507.

Bourgeault, Ivy, and Margaret MacDonald. 2000. "The Politics of Representation: Doing and Writing 'Interested' Research on Midwifery." *Resources for Feminist Research* 28 (1–2): 151–7.

Branswell, Helen. 2007. "Top Health Official Calls *Maclean's* Article on HPV Vaccine Alarmist, Unbalanced." Canadian Press, 17 August 2007.

– 2008. "Only One Partner Is No Protection from HPV." *Globe and Mail*, 14 January 2008. https://www.theglobeandmail.com/life/only-one-partner-is-no-protection-from-hpv/article4093408.

– 2012. "HPV and Boys: Female Physicians Urge Provinces, Territories to Pay for HPV Vaccine for Boys." *Toronto Star*, 7 February 2012. https://www.thestar.com/life/health_wellness/2012/02/07/hpv_and_boys_female_physicians_urge_provinces_territories_to_pay_for_hpv_vaccine_for_boys.html.

– 2013a. "Obstetricians and Gynecologists Group Calls for HPV Vaccine for Boys." *Maclean's*, 25 April 2013. https://www.macleans.ca/news/obstetricians-and-gynecologists-group-calls-for-hpv-vaccine-for-boys.

– 2013b. "Quebec Decides to Reduce Number of HPV Vaccine Doses, Saying 2 Is Enough." *Global News*, 23 August 2013. https://globalnews.ca/news/798631/quebec-decides-to-reduce-number-of-hpv-vaccine-doses-saying-2-is-enough.

– 2015. "Giving Boys the HPV Vaccine Could Cut Health-Care Costs: Study." *Global News*, 13 April 2015. https://globalnews.ca/news/1934887/giving-boys-the-hpv-vaccine-could-cut-health-care-costs-study.

Braun, Lundy, and Ling Phoun. 2010. "HPV Vaccination Campaigns: Masking Uncertainty, Erasing Complexity." In *Three Shots at Prevention: The HPV Vaccine and the Politics of Medicine's Simple Solutions*, edited by Keith Wailoo, Julie Livingston, Steven Epstein, and Robert Aronowitz, 39–60. Baltimore: John Hopkins University Press.

British Columbia Health. 2017. "B.C. Extends Free HPV Coverage to Boys." News release, 6 January 2017. https://news.gov.bc.ca/releases/2017HLTH0003-000027.

Brown, Adalsteinn. 2018. "DLSPH Open: Ontario Transparency Legislation to Impact Researchers and Clinicians." Dalla Lana School of Public Health.

https://www.dlsph.utoronto.ca/2018/02/15/dlsph-open-ontario
-transparency-legislation-to-impact-researchers-and-clinicians.

Brown, Sally, Jeannie Shoveller, Cathy Chabot, and Anthony D. LaMontagne. 2013. "Risk, Resistance and the Neoliberal Agenda: Young People, Health and Well-Being in the UK, Canada and Australia." *Health, Risk & Society* 15 (4): 333–46. https://doi.org/10.1080/13698575.2013.796346.

Burchell, Ann, Francois Coutlée, Pierre-Paul Tellier, James Hanley, and Eduardo Franco. 2011. "Genital Transmission of Human Papillomavirus in Recently Formed Heterosexual Couples." *Journal of Infectious Disease* 204, no. 11 (December): 1723–9. https://doi.org/10.1093/infdis/jir644.

Bury, Michael. 1982. "Chronic Illness as a Biographical Disruption." *Sociology of Health and Illness* 4, no. 2 (July): 167–82. https://doi.org/10.1111/1467-9566.ep11339939.

Butler, Judith. (1990) 2007. *Gender Trouble: Feminism and the Subversion of Identity.* New York: Routledge. https://doi.org/10.4324/9780203824979.

– 2004. *Undoing Gender.* New York: Routledge. https://doi.org/10.4324/9780203499627.

– 2008. "An Account of Oneself." In *Judith Butler in Conversation: Analyzing the Texts and Talk of Everyday Life,* edited by Bronwyn Davies, 19–38. New York: Routledge. https://doi.org/10.4324/9780203941447.

Butler-Jones, David. 2007. "What Ever Happened to 'An Ounce of Prevention'?" Letter to the editor, *Globe and Mail,* 17 September 2007. https://www.theglobeandmail.com/news/national/whatever-happened-to-an-ounce-of-prevention/article1082482.

Cairney, Paul. 2012. *Understanding Public Policy: Theories and Issues.* New York: Palgrave Macmillan.

Canada AM. 2011. "Ending the Gender Bias on HPV Vaccination." 26 October 2011.

Canadian Centre for Policy Alternatives (CCPA). 2019. *Unfinished Business: A Parallel Report on Canada's Implementation of the Beijing Declaration and Platform for Action.* Ottawa: CCPA. https://policyalternatives.ca/publications/reports/unfinished-business.

Canadian Immunization Committee (CIC). 2007. *Recommendations on a Human Papillomavirus Immunization Program.* Ottawa: Queen's Printer. https://www.canada.ca/en/public-health/services/immunization/recommendations-on-a-human-papillomavirus-immunization-program.html.

– 2014. "Summary of Canadian Immunization Committee (CIC) Recommendations for HPV Immunization Programs." *Canadian Communicable Disease Report* 40, no. 8 (April). https://doi.org/10.14745/ccdr.v40i08a02.

Canadian Medical Association Journal (CMAJ). 2013. "News: SOGC Recommends HPV Vaccination for Boys." *CMAJ* 185, no. 9 (June): E399. https://doi.org/10.1503/cmaj.109-4495.

Canadian Press. 2007a. "Budget: Pharmacists Support Funding of Health Technology." 19 March 2007.

– 2007b. "Young Females Advised to Get HPV Vaccine." 31 January 2007.

– 2008. "Premier Scolds Board for Refusing HPV Vaccine." *CTVNews*, 4 June 2008. https://toronto.ctvnews.ca/premier-scolds-board-for-refusing-hpv-vaccine-1.300240.

– 2012. "Toronto's Public Health Expands HPV Vaccine Program." *National Post*, 18 September 2012. https://nationalpost.com/posted-toronto /torontos-public-health-department-expands-hpv-vaccine-program-for -teen-girls.

– 2015a. "B.C. Bishop Urges Chastity over HPV Vaccine." *Toronto Star*, 25 September 2015. https://www.thestar.com/news/canada/2015/09/25 /bc-bishop-urges-chastity-over-hpv-vaccine.html.

– 2015b. "Vaccinating Boys against HPV Would Cut Health-Care Costs by Preventing Mouth and Throat Cancers: Study." *National Post*, 13 April 2015. https://nationalpost.com/health/vaccinating-boys-against-hpv-would -cut-health-care-costs-by-preventing-mouth-and-throat-cancers-study.

– 2016a. "Ontario Expands HPV Vaccine Program to Gay, Bisexual Men." *Toronto Star*, 28 June 2016. https://www.thestar.com/news/canada/2016 /06/28/ontario-expands-hpv-vaccine-program-to-gay-bisexual-men.html.

– 2016b. "Ontario HPV Vaccine Program Expanded to Include Boys, Grade 7 Students." *CTVNews*, 22 April 2016. https://london.ctvnews.ca/ontario-hpv -vaccine-program-expanded-to-include-boys-grade-7-students-1.2870315.

Canadian Women's Health Network (CWHN). 2007. *HPV, Vaccines, and Gender: Policy Considerations*. Winnipeg: CWHN.

Canwest News Service. 2009. "HPV Vaccine Safe for Boys." *Edmonton Journal*, 5 January 2009.

Castel, Robert. 1991. "From Dangerousness to Risk." In *The Foucault Effect: Studies in Governmentality*, edited by Graham Burchell, Colin Gordon, and Peter Miller, 281–98. Chicago: University of Chicago Press.

CBC News. 2013. "P.E.I. Boys Offered HPV Vaccine." 19 April 2013. https:// www.cbc.ca/news/canada/prince-edward-island/p-e-i-boys-offered-hpv -vaccine-1.1339059.

– 2015. "HPV Vaccine Program Expanded to 'Vulnerable' Boys, Men Under 26 in BC." 7 July 2015. https://www.cbc.ca/news/canada/british-columbia /hpv-vaccine-program-expanded-to-vulnerable-boys-men-under-26-in-b-c -1.3141712.

– 2016. "Vaccinating Ontario Boys for HPV Will Help with 'Herd Immunity.'" 25 April 2016. https://www.cbc.ca/news/canada/sudbury/boys-free-hpv -vaccine-sudbury-1.3551887.

Centers for Disease Control and Prevention (CDC). 2012. "HPV Infection Fact Sheet." Last modified 12 April 2022. http://www.cdc.gov/std/hpv/stdfact -hpv.htm.

Colbert, Yvonne. 2015. "HPV Vaccine for Nova Scotia Boys Called 'Groundbreaking.'" *CBC News*, 13 April 2015. https://www.cbc.ca/news/canada/nova-scotia/hpv-vaccine-for-nova-scotia-boys-called-groundbreaking-1.3031169.

Comeau, Pauline. 2007. "Debate Begins over Public Funding for HPV Vaccine." *CMAJ* 176, no. 7 (March): 913–14. https://doi.org/10.1503/cmaj.070269.

Conference Board of Canada. n.d. "Education Skills: University Completion." Accessed 14 March 2023. https://www.conferenceboard.ca/hcp/university-completion-aspx.

Connell, Erin. 2010. "The HPV Vaccination Campaign: A Project of Moral Regulation in an Era of Biopolitics." *Canadian Journal of Sociology* 35, no. 1 (March): 63–82. https://doi.org/10.29173/cjs6689.

Constantine, Norman A., and Petra Jerman. 2007. "Acceptance of Human Papillomavirus Vaccination among California Parents of Daughters: A Representative Statewide Analysis." *Journal of Adolescent Health* 40, no. 2 (February): 108–15. https://doi.org/10.1016/j.jadohealth.2006.10.007.

Cotter, John. 2013. "HPV Vaccine: Alberta May Include Boys in Program." *Toronto Star*, 5 May 2013. https://www.thestar.com/news/canada/2013/05/05/hpv_vaccine_alberta_may_include_boys_in_program.html.

Cowan, James. 2008. "HPV Vaccine Prevents Genital Lesions in Men, Merck Study Claims." *National Post*, 14 November 2008.

Craven, Christa, and Dána-Ain Davis, eds. 2013. *Feminist Activist Ethnography: Counterpoints to Neoliberalism in North America*. Lanham, MD: Lexington Books.

Crenshaw, K. 1989. "Demarginalizing the Intersection of Race and Sex: A Black Feminist Critique of Antidiscrimination Doctrine, Feminist Theory and Antiracist Politics." *University of Chicago Legal Forum* 1989 (1): 138–67. https://chicagounbound.uchicago.edu/uclf/vol1989/iss1/8.

Crighton, E.J., C. Brown, J. Baxter, L. Lemyre, J.R. Masuda, and F. Ursitti. 2013. "Perceptions and Experiences of Environmental Health Risks among New Mothers: A Qualitative Study in Ontario, Canada." *Health, Risk & Society* 15 (4): 295–312. https://doi.org/10.1080/13698575.2013.796345.

CTVNews. 2010. "HPV Vaccine Approved for Young Males in Canada." 23 February 2010. https://www.ctvnews.ca/hpv-vaccine-approved-for-young-males-in-canada-1.486056.

Das, Veena. 2001. "Stigma, Contagion, Defect: Issues in the Anthropology of Public Health." Paper presented at the Stigma and Global Health: Developing a Research Agenda International Conference, Bethesda, MD, 5–7 September 2001.

Dean, Mitchell. 1999. "Risk, Calculable and Incalculable." In *Risk and Sociocultural Theory: New Directions and Perspectives*, edited by Deborah Lupton, 131–59. Cambridge: Cambridge University Press. https://doi.org/10.1017/CBO9780511520778.007.

Dekker, Anthony. 2006. "Fostering Acceptance of Human Papillomavirus Vaccines." *Journal of the American Osteopathic Association* 106 (1): S14–18.

Department of Finance. 2007. "Canada's New Government Takes an Important Step to Improve Women's Health." News release, 16 April 2007. https://www .canada.ca/en/news/archive/2007/04/canada-new-government-takes -important-step-improve-women-health.html.

Di Leonardo, Micaela. 1998. *Exotics at Home: Anthropologies, Others, American Modernity*. Chicago: University of Chicago Press.

Donohue and Roach. 2012. "Too Young for the HPV Vaccine?" *Windsor Star*, 17 October 2012.

Douglas, Mary. (1966) 2002. *Purity and Danger*. London: Routledge.

– 1992. *Risk and Blame: Essays in Cultural Theory*. London: Routledge.

English, Kathy. 2015. "Public Editor Criticizes the *Star*'s Gardasil Story." *Toronto Star*, 13 February 2015. https://www.thestar.com/opinion/public_editor /2015/02/13/public-editor-criticizes-the-stars-gardasil-story.html.

Epstein, Steven. 2010. "The Great Undiscussable: Anal Cancer, HPV and Gay Men's Health." In *Three Shots at Prevention: The HPV Vaccine and the Politics of Medicine's Simple Solutions*, edited by Keith Wailoo, Julie Livingston, Steven Epstein, and Robert Aronowitz, 61–90. Baltimore: Johns Hopkins University Press.

Epstein, Steven, and April N. Huff. 2010. "Sex, Science, and the Politics of Biomedicine: Gardasil in a Comparative Perspective." In *Three Shots at Prevention: The HPV Vaccine and the Politics of Medicine's Simple Solutions*, edited by Keith Wailoo, Julie Livingston, Steven Epstein, and Robert Aronowitz, 213–28. Baltimore: Johns Hopkins University Press.

Ewald, Francois. 1991. "Insurance and Risk." In *The Foucault Effect: Studies in Governmentality*, edited by Graham Burchell, Colin Gordon, and Peter Miller, 197–210. Chicago: University of Chicago Press.

Ferguson, Rob. 2016. "Ontario Expanding HPV Vaccination Program to Include Boys." *Toronto Star*, 21 April 2016. https://www.thestar.com/news /queenspark/2016/04/21/ontario-expanding-hpv-vaccination-program-to -include-boys.html.

Findlay, Tammy. 2019. "Revisiting GBA/GBA+: Innovations and Interventions." *Canadian Public Administration* 62, no. 3 (September): 520–5. https://doi .org/10.1111/capa.12341.

Flera, Augie, and Roger Maaka. 2010. "Indigeneity-Grounded Analysis (IGA) as Policy(-Making) Lens: New Zealand Models, Canadian Realities." *International Indigenous Policy Journal* 1 (1): 1–12. https://doi.org/10.18584 /iipj.2010.1.1.4.

Foucault, Michel. (1969) 1989. *The Archaeology of Knowledge*. London: Routledge.

– (1978) 1990. *The History of Sexuality: An Introduction*. New York: Vintage Books.

– 1987. "The Ethic of Care for the Self as a Practice of Freedom." In *The Final Foucault*, edited by James Bernauer and David Rasmussen, 1–20. Cambridge, MA: MIT Press.

– 1989. *The Birth of a Clinic.* London: Routledge.

– 1991. "Governmentality." In *The Foucault Effect: Studies in Governmentality*, edited by Graham Burchell, Colin Gordon, and Peter Miller, 87–104. Chicago: University of Chicago Press.

– 1994. "Two Lectures." In *Critique and Power: Recasting the Foucault/Habermas Debate*, edited by Michael Kelly, 17–46. Cambridge, MA: MIT Press.

– 1997. "On the Genealogy of Ethics: An Overview of Work in Progress." In *Ethics: Subjectivity and* Truth, edited by Paul Rabinow, 253–80. Vol. 1 of *Essential Works of Foucault, 1954–1984.* London: Penguin Books.

– 1999. *Abnormal: Lectures at the College de France, 1974–1975.* New York: Picador.

Fox, Maggie. 2008. "Merck-Sponsored Study Suggests HPV Vaccine Benefits Men Too." *Globe and Mail*, 14 November 2008.

Fox, Nick J. 1997. "Postmodern Reflections on 'Risk,' 'Hazards' and Life Choices." In *Risk and Sociocultural Theory: New Directions and Perspectives*, edited by Deborah Lupton, 12–33. Cambridge: Cambridge University Press. https://doi.org/10.1017/CBO9780511520778.002.

Franco, Eduardo L., Alexanra de Pokomand, Andrea R. Spence, Ann N. Burchell, Helen Trottier, Marie-Hélène Mayrand, and Susie Lau. 2007. "Vaccination against Human Papillomavirus." *CMAJ* 177, no. 12 (December): 1524–8. https://doi.org/10.1503/cmaj.1070120.

Fraser, Sara. 2016. "P.E.I. Urging More High-Risk Adults to Get HPV Vaccine." *CBC News*, 15 November 2016. https://www.cbc.ca/news/canada/prince -edward-island/pei-hpv-boys-girls-cancer-virus-adults-vaccine-1.3851764.

Fung-Kee-Fung, Michael, Barry Rosen, Joan Murphy, Diane Provencher, and Marie Plante. 2007. "HPV Vaccine: A New Era in Cervical Cancer Prevention." *Globe and Mail*, 11 September 2007. https://www .theglobeandmail.com/amp/opinion/hpv-vaccine-a-new-era-in-cervical -cancer-prevention/article725276.

Gabriel, Sandra. 2014. "Preventative Measures for HPV and Cervical Cancer." *National Post*, 8 March 2014.

Garro, Linda. 2000. "Cultural Knowledge as Resource in Illness Narratives: Remembering through Accounts of Illness." In *Narrative and the Cultural Construction of Illness and Healing*, edited by Cheryl Mattingly and Linda Garro, 70–87. Berkeley: University of California Press.

Giddens, Anthony. 1991. *Modernity and Self-Identity: Self and Society in the Late Modern Age.* Cambridge: Polity Press.

Gillespie, Kerry. 2007. "Ads for HPV Vaccine Yanked." *Toronto Star*, 18 September 2007. http://www.thestar.com/ontarioelection/article/257699.

Gilman, Marina, Sander L. Gilman, and Michael M. Johns III. 2009. "Human Papillomavirus, Abstinence, and the Other Risks." *The Lancet* 373, no. 9673 (April): 1420–1. https://doi.org/10.1016/S0140-6736(09)60810-2.

Ginn, Diana. 2004. "The Supreme Court of Canada and What It Means to Be 'Of Woman Born.'" In *From Motherhood to Mothering: The Legacy of Adrienne Rich's Of Woman Born*, edited by Andrea O'Reilly, 27–43. Albany: State University of New York Press.

Giroux, Henry. 2010. *Youth in a Suspect Society: Democracy or Disposability?* New York: Palgrave Macmillan.

Glenn, Evelyn N. 1994. "Social Constructions of Mothering: A Thematic Overview." In *Mothering: Ideology, Experience, and Agency*, edited by Evelyn N. Glenn, Grace Chang, and Linda R. Forcey, 1–29. New York: Routledge. https://doi.org/10.4324/9781315538891.

Globe and Mail. 2007. "Saving Women's Lives." Editorial, 21 September 2007.

Goffman, Erving. 1963. *Stigma: Notes on the Management of Spoiled Identity*. New York: Simon & Schuster.

Gold, Ronald. 2015. "Vaccine's 'Dark Side' Overstated." Letter to the editor, *Toronto Star*, 14 February 2015. https://www.thestar.com/opinion/letters _to_the_editors/2015/02/14/vaccines-dark-side-overstated.html.

Gordon, Andrea. 2009. "Gardasil® Side Effects Examined: HPV Vaccine Causes Some Adverse Reactions, U.S. Study Confirms." *Toronto Star*, 19 August 2009, E1.

Gordon, Colin. 1991. "Government Rationality: An Introduction." In *The Foucault Effect: Studies in Governmentality*, edited by Graham Burchell, Colin Gordon, and Peter Miller, 1–52. Chicago: University of Chicago Press.

Government of Canada. 2007. *House of Commons Debates*. Vol. 141, Number 134, 1st Session, 39th Parliament, 17 April 2007. Ottawa: House of Commons Canada. https://www.ourcommons.ca/DocumentViewer/en/39-1/house /sitting-134/hansard.

Government of Ontario. 2017a. "Getting the HPV Vaccine." Last modified 21 October 2021. http://www.health.gov.on.ca/en/ms/hpv.

– 2017b. Health Sector Payment Transparency Act, 2017, S.O. 2017, c. 25, Sched. 4. https://www.ontario.ca/laws/statute/17h25.

– 2021. "Ontario Taking Action to Protect against Omicron Variant: Vaccines Remain Best Defence against COVID-19 and Variants." News release, 10 December 2021. https://news.ontario.ca/en/release/1001327/ontario -taking-action-to-protect-against-omicron-variant.

Government of Quebec. n.d. "Human Papillomavirus (HPV) Vaccination Program." Last modified 17 January 2023. https://www.quebec.ca/en /health/advice-and-prevention/vaccination/human-papillomavirus-hpv -vaccination-program/history-of-the-program.

Government of Saskatchewan. 2017. "Human Papillomavirus Vaccine." Fact
sheet, 9 August 2017. https://pubsaskdev.blob.core.windows.net
/pubsask-prod/76359/76359-HPV-9_August_2017.pdf.

Graham, Janice. 2005. "Smart Regulation: Will the Government's Strategy
Work?" *CMAJ* 173, no. 12 (December): 1469–70. https://doi.org/10.1503
/cmaj.050424.

Grant, Kelly. 2018. "Ontario Law to Require Drug Firms to Reveal Funds Paid
to Doctor's Groups, Patient Advocates." *Globe and Mail*, 22 February 2018.
https://www.theglobeandmail.com/news/national/ontario-law-to
-require-drug-firms-to-reveal-funds-paid-to-doctors-groups-patient-advocates
/article38061619.

Graveland, Bill. 2009. "HPV Vaccine a Tough Sell in Parts of Canada;
Vaccination Rates High in Quebec." *Winnipeg Free Press*, 2 March 2009. https://
www.winnipegfreepress.com/arts-and-life/life/health/2009/03/02/hpv
-vaccine-a-tough-sell-in-parts-of-canada-vaccination-rates-high-in-quebec.

Greaves, Lorraine. 2009. "Women, Gender, and Health Research." In *Women's
Health: Intersections of Policy, Research and Practice*, edited by Pat Armstrong and
Jennifer Deadman, 3–20. Toronto: Women's Press.

Gregg, Jessica. 2003. *Virtually Virgins: Sexual Strategies and Cervical Cancer in
Recife, Brazil*. Stanford, CA: Stanford University Press.

– 2011. "An Unanticipated Source of Hope: Stigma and Cervical Cancer in
Brazil." *Medical Anthropology Quarterly* 25, no. 1 (March): 70–84. https://doi.org
/10.1111/j.1548-1387.2010.01137.x.

Greslé-Favier, Claire. 2006. "Pro-abstinence Discourses and the Definition
of the Conservative Identity in the Contemporary United States." *Current
Objectives of Postgraduate American Studies* 7:1–6. http://dx.doi.org/10.5283
/copas.91.

Griffith, Janessa, Husayn Marani, and Helen Monkman. 2021. "COVID-19
Vaccine Hesitancy in Canada: Content Analysis of Tweets Using the
Theoretical Domains Framework." *Journal of Medical Internet Research* 23, no. 4
(April): e26874. https://doi.org/10.2196/26874.

Gross, Sky E., and Judith T. Shuval. 2008. "On Knowing and Believing: Prenatal
Genetic Screening and Resistance to 'Risk Medicine.'" *Health, Risk & Society*
10 (6): 549–64. https://doi.org/10.1080/13698570802533721.

Guelph Mercury. 2007. "HPV Vaccine Needed because Some Cervical Cancers
Hard to Treat, Researcher Says." 20 October 2007.

Guichon, Juliet, and Rupert Kaul. 2015. "Science Shows HPV Vaccine Has No
Dark Side." *Toronto Star*, 11 February 2015. Last modified 23 December 2015.
https://www.thestar.com/opinion/commentary/2015/02/11/science
-shows-hpv-vaccine-has-no-dark-side.html.

Gulli, Cathy. 2007. "Our Girls Are Not Guinea Pigs: Is an Upcoming Mass
Inoculation of a Generation Unnecessary and Potentially Dangerous?"

Macleans, 23 August 2007. https://archive.macleans.ca/article/2007/8/27
/our-girls-are-not-guinea-pigs.

Ha, Tu Thanh. 2008. "Allergy to HPV Vaccine Is Rare, but Still Dangerous,
Australian Study Finds." *Globe and Mail,* 2 September 2008. https://www
.theglobeandmail.com/life/allergy-to-hpv-vaccine-is-rare-but-still-dangerous
-australian-study-finds/article17971262.

Hamilton Spectator. 2007. "HPV Vaccine Urged for Girls 9 to 13." 1 February 2007.

Hankivsky, Olena. 2007a. "Engendering Evidence: Transforming Economic
Evaluations." In *Women's Health in Canada: Critical Perspectives on Theory and
Policy,* edited by Marina Morrow, Olena Hankivsky, and Colleen Varcoe,
169–95. Toronto: University of Toronto Press.

– 2007b. "Gender-Based Analysis and Health Policy: The Need to Rethink
Outdated Strategies." In *Women's Health in Canada: Critical Perspectives on
Theory and Policy,* edited by Marina Morrow, Olena Hankivsky, and Colleen
Varcoe, 143–68. Toronto: University of Toronto Press.

– 2012a. "The Lexicon of Mainstreaming Equality: Gender Based Analysis
(GBA), Gender and Diversity Analysis (GDA) and Intersectionality Based
Analysis (IBA)." *Canadian Political Science Review* 6 (2–3): 171–83. https://
ojs.unbc.ca/index.php/cpsr/article/view/278.

– 2012b. "Women's Health, Men's Health, and Gender and Health:
Implications for Intersectionality." *Social Science & Medicine* 74, no. 11 (June):
1712–20. https://doi.org/10.1016/j.socscimed.2011.11.029.

Hankivsky, Olena, and Renée Cormier. 2009. *Intersectionality: Moving Women's
Health Research and Policy Forward.* Vancouver: Women's Health Research
Network. https://cewh.ca/wp-content/uploads/2012/05/2009
_IntersectionaliyMovingwomenshealthresearchandpolicyforward.pdf.

Hankivsky, Olena, and Linda Mussell. 2018. "Gender-Based Analysis Plus in
Canada: The Problems and Possibilities of Integrating Intersectionality."
Canadian Public Policy 44, no. 4 (December): 303–16. https://doi.org/10
.3138/cpp.2017-058.

Hanson, Barbara. 2000. "The Social Construction of Sex Categories as
Problematic to Biomedical Research: Cancer as a Case in Point." In *Health,
Illness, and Use of Care: The Impact of Social Factors,* edited by Jennie Jacobs
Kronenfeld, 53–68. Bingley, UK: Emerald Group Publishing. https://doi
.org/10.1016/S0275-4959(00)80022-8.

Hayes, Sharon. 1996. *The Cultural Contradictions of Motherhood.* New Haven, CT:
Yale University Press.

Health Canada. 2000. *Health Canada's Gender-Based Analysis Policy.* Ottawa: Minister
of Public Works and Government Services Canada. https://publications.gc.ca
/collections/Collection/H34-110-2000E.pdf.

– 2003a. *Exploring Concepts of Gender and Health.* Ottawa: Women's Health Bureau.
https://publications.gc.ca/collections/Collection/H21-216-2003E.pdf.

– 2003b. "Healthy Living: Gender-Based Analysis." Accessed 11 February 2012.
http://.hc-sc.gc.ca/hl-vs/pubs/womenfemmes/gender-sexes-eng.php (site
discontinued).

– 2006. "Notice of Decision for Gardasil. Accessed 3 March 2020. http://www
.hcsc.gc.ca/dhp-mps/prodpharma/sbd-smd/phase!-decision/drug-med
/nd_ad_2006_Gardasil®_102682-eng.php (site discontinued).

– 2007. "Summary Basis of Decision (SBD) for GARDASIL™." Last modified
14 July 2021. https://hpr-rps.hres.ca/reg-content/summary-basis-decision
-detailOne.php?lang=en&linkID=SBD00066.

HealthLink BC. 2017. "Human Papillomavirus (HPV) Vaccines." Last modified
1 June 2022. https://www.healthlinkbc.ca/healthlinkbc-files/hpv-vaccines.

HealthSOGC. 2016. "HPV – You Could Be at Risk." YouTube video, 0:15.
14 October 2016. https://www.youtube.com/watch?v=ACF6a8E4AVI
&feature=youtube.

Henry, Frances, and Carol Tator. 2002. *Discourses of Domination: Racial Bias in
the Canadian English-Language Press.* Toronto: University of Toronto Press.
https://doi.org/10.3138/9781442673946.

Henry, Fred. 2008. "Does Vaccine Turn Girls into Guinea Pigs?" Letter to the
editor, *Calgary Herald*, 28 October 2008, A13.

– 2012. "HPV Vaccine Supporters Aren't Doctors of the Soul." Letter to the
editor, *Calgary Herald*, 27 June 2012, A15.

Herskovits, Beth. 2007. "Brand of the Year." *Pharmaceutical Executive* 7 (2):
60–70. https://www.pharmexec.com/view/brand-year-0.

H. Krueger and Associates. 2008. *Implementing a Human Papillomavirus
Vaccination Program: Evidence on Cost-Effectiveness.* Delta, BC: H. Krueger and
Associates.

Hobson-West, Tru. 2010. "Understanding Vaccination Resistance: Moving
Beyond Risk." *Health, Risk & Society* 5 (3): 273–83. https://doi.org/10.1080
/13698570310001606978.

Holzer, Boris, and Mads P. Sørensen. 2003. "Rethinking Subpolitics: Beyond the
'Iron Cage' of Modern Politics?" *Theory, Culture & Society* 20, no. 2 (April):
79–102. https://doi.org/10.1177/0263276403020002005.

Hughes, Rachel. 2003. "The Abject Artifacts of Memory: Photographs from
Cambodia's Genocide." *Media, Culture & Society* 25, no. 1 (January): 23–44.
https://doi.org/10.1177/0163443703025001632.

Hunt, Linda. 2000. "Strategic Suffering: Illness Narratives as Social
Empowerment among Mexican Cancer Patients." In *Narrative and the Cultural
Construction of Illness and Healing,* edited by Cheryl Mattingly and Linda
Garro, 88–107. Berkeley: University of California Press.

Inhorn, Marcia. 2006. "Defining Women's Health: A Dozen Messages from
More than 150 Ethnographers." *Medical Anthropology Quarterly* 20, no. 3
(September): 345–78. https://doi.org/10.1525/maq.2006.20.3.345.

Jackson, Beth, Ann Pederson, and Madeline Boscoe. 2009. "Waiting to Wait: Improving Wait Times Evidence through Gender-Based Analysis." In *Women's Health: Intersections of Policy, Research and Practice*, edited by Pat Armstrong and Jennifer Deadman, 35–51. Toronto: Women's Press.

Jacobson, Robert M., Paul V. Targonski, and Gregory A. Poland. 2007. "A Taxonomy of Reasoning Flaws in the Anti-vaccine Movement." *Vaccine* 25, no. 16 (April): 3146–52. https://doi.org/10.1016/j.vaccine.2007.01.046.

Jaslow, Ryan. 2013. "Katie Couric Admits Disproportionate Reporting on HPV Vaccine Controversy." *CBS News*, 10 December 2013. https://www.cbsnews.com/news/katie-couric-hpv-vaccine-show-criticism-valid.

Kaufert, Patricia. 2000. "Screening the Body: The Pap Smear and the Mammogram." In *Living and Working with the New Medical Technologies: Intersections of Inquiry*, edited by Margaret Lock, Allan Young, and Alberto Cambrosio, 165–83. Cambridge: Cambridge University Press.

Keenan, Tom. 2007. "Boys Can't Escape Reach of Infection: The Debate about Vaccinating Girls against HPV Has Too Often Ignored the Role of Males." *Calgary Herald*, 8 March 2007

Keniston, Ann. 2004. "Beginning with 'I': The Legacy of Adrienne Rich's *Of Woman Born*." In *From Motherhood to Mothering: The Legacy of Adrienne Rich's* Of Woman Born, edited by Andrea O'Reilly, 223–40. Albany: State University of New York Press.

Kirkey, Sharon. 2007. "Young Girls Require Vaccine, Panel Says: Virus Spread through Sex Causes Cervical Cancer." *National Post*, 31 January 2007, A1.

– 2014. "Increase in HPV-Tied Cancers 'Disturbing': Researchers." *Vancouver Sun*, 23 July 2014, B2.

Kirmayer, Laurence. 2000. "Broken Narratives: Clinical Encounters and the Poetics of Illness Experience." In *Narrative and the Cultural Construction of Illness and Healing*, edited by Cheryl Mattingly and Linda Garro, 153–80. Berkeley: University of California Press.

Kleinman, Arthur. 1988. *The Illness Narratives: Suffering, Healing, and the Human Condition*. New York: Basic Books.

Kohler Riessman, Catherine. 2000. "'Even If We Don't Have Children [We] Can Live': Stigma and Infertility in South India." In *Narrative and the Cultural Construction of Illness and Healing*, edited by Cheryl Mattingly and Linda Garro, 128–52. Berkeley: University of California Press.

Kraicer-Melamed Hannah, and Caroline Quach. 2017. "Expanding Free School-Based Human Papilloma Virus (HPV) Vaccination Programs to Include School-Aged Males in Nova Scotia, Canada." *Health Reform Observer/Observatoire des Réformes de Santé* 5 (2). https://doi.org/10.13162/hro-ors.v5i2.2851.

Kubacki, Maria. 2007. "Pediatricians Group Backs HPV Vaccine for Girls; Recommends Shot for Nine- to 13-Year-Olds." *Ottawa Citizen*, 25 September 2007.

Laucius, Joanne. 2007a. "Doctors Call for Use of HPV Vaccine." *Vancouver Sun*, 21 June 2007.

– 2007b. "HPV Vaccine Under Fire; Medical Journal Raises Questions about Treatment that 'Prevents' Cervical Cancer." *Calgary Herald*, 2 August 2007.

Lawrence, Susan C., and Kae Bendixen. 1992. "His and Hers: Male and Female Anatomy in Anatomy Texts for U.S. Medical Students, 1890–1989." *Social Science & Medicine* 35, no. 7 (October): 925–34. https://doi.org/10.1016 /0277-9536(92)90107-2.

Lear, Dana. 1995. "Sexual Communication in the Age of AIDS: The Construction of Risk and Trust among Young Adults." *Social Science & Medicine* 41, no. 9 (November): 1311–23. https://doi.org/10.1016/0277 -9536(95)00010-5.

Ledford, Heidi. 2021. "COVID Vaccines and Blood Clots: What Researchers Know So Far." *Nature*, 24 August 2021. https://www.nature.com/articles /d41586-021-02291-2.

Leiss, William, Stephen Kline, and Sut Jhally. 1990. *Social Communication in Advertising: Persons, Products and Images of Well-Being*. Scarborough, ON: Nelson.

Lerner, Andrea M., Gregory K. Folkers, and Anthony S. Fauci. 2020. "Preventing the Spread of SARS-CoV-2 with Masks and Other 'Low-Tech' Interventions." *JAMA* 324, no. 19 (October): 1935–6. https://doi.org/10 .1001/jama.2020.21946.

Leung, Wendy. 2012. "Why Some Parents Still Won't Give Daughters the HPV Vaccine." *Globe and Mail*, 16 October 2012. https://www.theglobeandmail .com/life/health-and-fitness/health/why-some-parents-still-wont-give -daughters-the-hpv-vaccine/article4616841.

Lexchin, Joel. 1999. "Hear No Secrets, See No Secrets, Speak No Secrets: Secrecy in the Canadian Drug Approval System." *International Journal of Social Determinants of Health and Health Services* 29, no. 1 (January): 167–78. https://doi.org/10.2190/RM7E-748K-K4XM -HHQP.

Lieber, Eugene. 2009. "Faith and Logic." Letter to the editor, *Edmonton Journal*, 17 January 2009.

Lieblich, Amia, Rivka Tuval-Mashiach, and Tamar Zilber. 1998. *Narrative Research: Reading, Analysis and Interpretation*. Thousand Oaks, CA: Sage Publications.

Lippman, Abby. 2007. "Bigger Problem." Letter to the editor, *Ottawa Citizen*, 21 March 2007.

Lippman, Abby, Ryan Melnychuk, Carolyn Shimmin, and Madeline Boscoe. 2007. "Human Papillomavirus, Vaccines and Women's Health: Questions and Cautions." *CMAJ* 177, no. 5 (August): 484–7. https://doi.org/10.1503 /cmaj.070944.

Lock, Margaret, and Judith Farquhar. 2007. "Introduction." In *Beyond the Body Proper: Reading the Anthropology of Material Life*, edited by Margaret Lock and Judith Farquhar, 1–16. Durham, NC: Duke University Press.

Lock, Margaret, and Patricia Kaufert. 1998. "Introduction." In *Pragmatic Women and Body Politics*, edited by Margaret Lock and Patricia Kaufert, 1–27. Cambridge: Cambridge University Press.

Lopez-Leon, Sandra, Talia Wegman-Ostrosky, Carol Perelman, Rosalinda Sepulveda, Paulina A. Robolledo, Angelica Cuapio, and Sonia Villapol. 2021. "More Than 50 Long-Term Effects of COVID-19: A Systematic Review and Meta-Analysis." *Scientific Reports* 11:16144. https://doi.org/10.1038/s41598-021-95565-8.

Lupton, Deborah. 1994. *Medicine as Culture: Illness, Disease and the Body in Western Societies*. London: Sage Publications.

– 1995. *The Imperative of Health: Public Health and the Regulated Body*. London: Sage Publications.

– 1999a. "Introduction: Risk and Sociocultural Theory." In *Risk and Sociocultural Theory: New Directions and Perspectives*, edited by Deborah Lupton, 1–11. Cambridge: Cambridge University Press. https://doi.org/10.1017/CBO9780511520778.001.

– 1999b. "Risk and the Ontology of Pregnant Embodiment." In *Risk and Sociocultural Theory: New Directions and Perspectives*, edited by Deborah Lupton, 59–85. Cambridge: Cambridge University Press. https://doi.org/10.1017/CBO9780511520778.004.

– 2003. *Medicine as Culture*. 2nd ed. London: Sage Publication.

Lupton, Deborah, and Alan Petersen. 1996. *The New Public Health: Health and Self in the Age of Risk*. London: Sage Publications. https://dx.doi.org/10.4135/9781446217429.

MacKinnon, Bobbi-Jean. 2017. "A 'No-Brainer': N.B. Medical Community Welcomes HPV Vaccine for Boys." *CBC News*, 19 February 2017. https://www.cbc.ca/news/canada/new-brunswick/hpv-vaccine-boys-cancer-new-brunswick-1.3983937.

MacLeod, Meredith. 2013. "Halton Catholic Schools to Offer HPV Shots." *Toronto Star*, 5 November 2013. https://www.thestar.com/yourtoronto/education/2013/11/05/halton_catholic_schools_to_offer_hpv_shots.html.

Mah, Catherine L., Raisa B. Deber, Astrid Guttmann, Allison McGeer, and Murray Krahn. 2011. "Another Look at the Human Papillomavirus Vaccine Experience in Canada." *American Journal of Public Health* 101, no. 10 (October): 1850–7. https://doi.org/10.2105/AJPH.2011.300205.

Mai, Verna. 2007. "The HPV Vaccine Is about Preventing Cancer. Period." *Toronto Star*, 21 September 2007. https://www.thestar.com/opinion/2007/09/21/the_hpv_vaccine_is_about_preventing_cancer_period.html.

Mallick, Heather. 2015. "Vaccine Debate Is One We Shouldn't Even Be Having." *Toronto Star*, 6 February 2015. https://www.thestar.com/news/canada /2015/02/06/vaccine-debate-is-one-we-shouldnt-even-be-having-mallick .html.

Manitoba Health. 2017. *Manitoba's HPV Immunization Program: Questions and Answers for Health Care Providers*. Winnipeg: Manitoba Health. http://www .gov.mb.ca/health/publichealth/cdc/docs/hpv_phn_qa.pdf.

Mansi, James. 2008. "Gardasil Is as Safe as Any Other Vaccine." Letter to the editor, *Edmonton Journal*, 5 October 2008.

– 2009. "Gardasil Is Safe." Letter to the editor, *National Post*, 2 June 2009.

Marcus, George E. 2009. "Introduction: Notes Toward an Ethnographic Memoir of Supervising Graduate Research through Anthropology's Decades of Transformation." In *Fieldwork is Not What It Used to Be: Learning Anthropology's Method in a Time of Transition*, edited by James D. Faubion and George E. Marcus, 1–31. Ithaca, NY: Cornell University Press. https://www .jstor.org/stable/10.7591/j.ctt7zfjh.4.

Martin, Emily. 2007. "The Egg and the Sperm: How Science Has Constructed a Romance Based on Stereotypical Male-Female Roles." In *Beyond the Body Proper: Reading the Anthropology of Material Life*, edited by Margaret Lock and Judith Farquar, 417–27. Durham, NC: Duke University Press.

McClure, Kirstie. 1992. "The Issue of Foundations: Scientized Politics, Politicized Science, and Feminist Critical Practice." In *Feminists Theorize the Political*, edited by Judith Butler and Joan W. Scott, 341–68. New York: Routledge.

McGregor, Glen. 2007. "Worst-Kept Secret: Former PM Advisor Manning Tory War Room." *Ottawa Citizen*, 12 April 2007.

Merck Frosst. 2011a. "Health Canada Approves Gardasil®9 (Human Papillomavirus 9-Valent Vaccine, Recombinant) for the Prevention of Oropharyngeal and Other Head and Neck Cancers." News release, 11 April 2011. https://www.newswire.ca/news-releases/health-canada-approves -gardasil-r-9-human-papillomavirus-9-valent-vaccine-recombinant-for-the -prevention-of-oropharyngeal-and-other-head-and-neck-cancers-812857465. html.

– 2011b. "New England Journal of Medicine Publishes Efficacy and Safety Data for Gardasil® in Males." News release, 26 October 2011. https://www.merck .com/news/new-england-journal-of-medicine-publishes-additional-efficacy -and-safety-data-for-gardasil-in-males.

– 2015. "Merck's HPV Vaccine, Gardasil®9, Now Available in Canada." News release, 1 April 2015. https://www.newswire.ca/news-releases/mercks-hpv -vaccine-gardasil9-now-available-in-canada-517470221.html.

Mintzes, Barbara. 2010. "'Ask Your Doctor': Women and Direct-to-Consumer Advertising." In *The Push to Prescribe: Women and Canadian Drug Policy*, edited by Anne Rochon Ford and Diane Saibil, 17–46. Toronto: Women's Press.

Montreal Gazette. 2007. "Vaccine Program the Right Move." Editorial, 26 September 2007.

– 2014. "Make HPV Vaccines Available for Boys in Schools." Editorial, 26 July 2014, B6.

Moore, Sarah E.H. 2010. "Is the Healthy Body Gendered? Toward a Feminist Critique of the New Paradigm of Health." *Body & Society* 16, no. 2 (June): 95–118. https://doi.org/10.1177/1357034X10364765.

Morrison, Ken. 1995. *Marx, Durkheim, Weber: Formations of Modern Social Thought.* London: Sage Publications.

Mule, Nick J. 2020. "State Involvement in LGBT+ Health and Social Support Issues in Canada." *International Journal of Environmental Research and Public Health* 17, no. 19 (October): 7314. https://doi.org/10.3390/ijerph17197314.

Munoz, Nubia, Xavier Castellsague, Amy Berrington de Gonzalez, and Lutz Gissman. 2006. "Chapter 1: HPV in the Etiology of Human Cancer." *Vaccine* 24, no. S3 (August): S1–10. https://doi.org/10.1016/j.vaccine.2006.05.115.

Murphy, Joan. 2008. "Benefits of HPV Vaccine Outweigh Risks." *Toronto Star*, 3 November 2008. https://www.thestar.com/opinion/2008/11/03/benefits _of_hpv_vaccine_outweigh_risk.html.

National Advisory Committee on Immunization (NACI). 2007. *Statement on Human Papillomavirus Vaccine.* Ottawa: Public Health Agency of Canada. https://www.canada.ca/content/dam/phac-aspc/migration/phac-aspc /publicat/ccdr-rmtc/07pdf/acs33-02.pdf.

– 2012. *Update on Human Papillomavirus (HPV) Vaccines.* Ottawa: Public Health Agency of Canada. https://doi.org/10.14745/ccdr.v38i00a01.

– 2015. *Update on the Recommended Human Papillomavirus (HPV) Vaccine Immunization Schedule.* Ottawa: Public Health Agency of Canada. https://www .canada.ca/content/dam/canada/public-health/migration/publications /healthy-living-vie-saine/papillomavirus-immunization-schedule-2015 -papillome-immunisation-calendrier/alt/papillomavirus-immunization -schedule-papillome-immunisation-calendrier-eng.pdf.

– 2017. *Updated Recommendations on Human Papillomavirus (HPV) Vaccines: 9-Valent HPV Vaccine 2-Dose Immunization Schedule and the Use of Vaccines in Immunocompromised Individuals.* Ottawa: Public Health Agency of Canada. https://www.canada.ca/content/dam/phac-aspc/documents/services /publications/healthy-living/updated-recommendations-human -papillomavirus-immunization-schedule-immunocompromised-populations /updated-recommendations-human-papillomavirus-immunization-schedule -immunocompromised-populationsv3-eng.pdf.

– 2021. *An Advisory Committee Statement (ACS) National Advisory Committee on Immunization (NACI) Guidance on Booster COVID-19 Vaccine Doses in Canada –Update December 3, 2021.* Ottawa: Public Health Agency of Canada. https://www.canada.ca/content/dam/phac-aspc/documents/services /immunization/national-advisory-committee-on-immunization-naci/guidance -booster-covid-19-vaccine-doses/guidance-booster-covid-19-vaccine-doses.pdf.

National Cancer Institute. 2012. "HPV and Cancer." Last modified 12
  September 2012. http://www.cancer.gov/cancertopics/factsheet/Risk
  /HPV.
National Post. 2015. "Preventing HPV in Males Would Save Lives – And Money."
  Editorial, 22 April 2015. https://nationalpost.com/opinion/national
  -post-view-preventing-hpv-in-males-would-save-lives-and-money.
Native Women's Association of Canada (NWAC). 2007. *Culturally Relevant
  Gender Based Analysis: An Issue Paper.* Corner Brook, NL: NWAC. https://www
  .nwac.ca/assets-knowledge-centre/2007-NWAC-Culturally-Relevant
  -Gender-Based-Analysis-An-Issue-Paper.pdf.
Nealon, Joshua, and Benjamin J. Cowling. 2022. "Omicron Severity: Milder
  but Not Mild." *The Lancet* 399, no. 10323 (January): 412–13. https://doi
  .org/10.1016/S0140-6736(22)00056-3.
Nettleton, Sarah. 1996. "Women and the New Paradigm of Health and
  Medicine." *Critical Social Policy* 16, no. 33 (August): 33–53. https://doi.org
  /10.1177/026101839601604802.
– 1997. "Governing the Risky Self: How to Become Healthy, Wealthy and Wise."
  In *Foucault: Health and Medicine*, edited by Robin Bunton and Alan Petersen,
  207–22. New York: Routledge.
Office of the Commissioner of Lobbying of Canada. 2007a. "Registration – In-
  House Corporation: Merck Canada Inc. (2007-05-30 to 2007-10-30)."
  Registry of Lobbyists. Last modified 22 November 2022. https://
  lobbycanada.gc.ca
  /app/secure/ocl/lrs/do/vwRg?cno=12241&regId=506154#regStart.
– 2007b. "Registration – In-House Corporation: Merck Canada Inc. (2007-10-30
  to 2008-05-21)." Registry of Lobbyists. Last modified 22 November 2022.
  https://lobbycanada.gc.ca/app/secure/ocl/lrs/do/vwRg?cno=12241
  &regId=510147#regStart.
– 2008. "Registration – In-House Corporation: Merck Canada Inc. (2008-
  05-21 to 2008-07-08)." Registry of Lobbyists. Last modified 22 November
  2022. https://lobbycanada.gc.ca/app/secure/ocl/lrs/do/vwRg?cno=12241
  &regId=514495#regStart.
Office of the Premier (Ontario). 2007. "McGuinty Government Launches
  Life-Saving HPV Immunization Program: New, Free Vaccines to Be Offered
  to Young Women in Grade Eight this Fall." News release, 2 August 2007.
  https://news.ontario.ca/en/release/3863/mcguinty-government-launches
  -life-saving-hpv-immunization-program.
Olshen, Elyse, Elizabeth R. Woods, S. Bryn Austin, Marlise Luskin, and Howard
  Bauchner. 2005. "Parental Acceptance of the Human Papillomavirus
  Vaccine." *Journal of Adolescent Health* 37, no. 3 (September): 248–51. https://
  doi.org/10.1016/j.jadohealth.2005.05.016.
O'Malley, Kadey. 2007. "Meet North America's Most Contentious Vaccine."
  Macleans, 21 March 2007.

O'Reilly, Andrea. 2004a. "Introduction." In *From Motherhood to Mothering: The Legacy of Adrienne Rich's* Of Woman Born, edited by Andrea O'Reilly, 1–23. Albany: State University of New York Press.

– 2004b. "Introduction." In *Mother Outlaws: Theories and Practices of Empowered Mothering*, edited by Andrea O'Reilly, 1–28. Toronto: Women's Press.

– 2010. "Outlaw(ing) Motherhood: A Theory and Politic of Maternal Empowerment for the Twenty-First Century." In *Twenty-First-Century Motherhood: Experience, Identity, Policy, Agency*, edited by Andrea O'Reilly, 366–80. New York: Columbia University Press.

Ortner, Sherry. 1974. "Is Female to Male as Nature Is to Culture?" In *Women, Culture, and Society*, edited by Michelle Rosaldo and Louise Lamphere, 67–87. Stanford, CA: Stanford University Press.

O'Sullivan, Tracey, and Carol Amaratunga. 2009. "Women in the Response Community: Gendered Impacts of Bio-disasters." In *Women's Health: Intersections of Policy, Research and Practice*, edited by Pat Armstrong and Jennifer Deadman, 217–31. Toronto: Women's Press.

Owens, Brian. 2019. "Ontario Delays Implementation of Pharma Transparency Rules." *CMAJ News*, 6 February 2019. https://cmajnews.com/2019/02/06 /ontario-delays-implementation-of-pharma-transparency-rules-cmaj-109-5718.

Page, Shelley. 2007a. "Everything You Wanted to Know, but Were Afraid to Ask: Is the HPV Vaccine a Victory for Women's Health or the Triumph of Aggressive Marketing?" *Ottawa Citizen*, 29 April 2007, B5.

– 2007b. "To Market a Drug; Financing a Vaccine against Cervical Cancer May Be the Right Thing to Do, but a Multinational Giant's Aggressive Campaign Has Muddied the Debate." *Vancouver Sun*, 14 May 2007, A11.

Pandolfi, Mariella. 2007. "Memory within the Body: Women's Narrative and Identity in a Southern Italian Village." In *Beyond the Body Proper: Reading the Anthropology of Material Life*, edited by Margaret Lock and Judith Farquhar, 451–8. Durham, NC: Duke University Press.

Paoletti, Jo B. 1997. "The Gendering of Infant's and Toddler's Clothing." In *The Material Culture of Gender/The Gender of Material Culture*, edited by Katherine Martinez and Kenneth L. Ames, 27–35. Winterhur, DE: Henry Francis du Pont Museum.

Parkin, D. Maxwell, and Freddie Bray. 2006. "Chapter 2: The Burden of HPV-Related Cancers." *Vaccine* 25, no. 3 (August): S11–25. https://doi.org/10 .1016/j.vaccine.2006.05.111.

Parks, Michelle, and David A. Salisbury. 2007. "HPV Vaccine Underwent Rigorous Analysis." *Ottawa Citizen*, 6 December 2007, A13.

Peirson, Mary. 2008. "Parents and HPV Vaccine." Letter to the editor, *Globe and Mail*, 22 April 2008. https://www.theglobeandmail.com/opinion/letters /parents-and-hpv-vaccine/article958932.

Pellizzari, Rosana. 2012. "Why Wouldn't You Protect Your Kids?" Letter to the editor, *Peterborough Examiner*, 15 August 2012.

Peres, Judy. 2010. "Who Should Get the HPV Vaccine? Usage Expands Amid Debate." *JNCI: Journal of the National Cancer Institute* 102, no. 12 (June): 838–40. https://doi.org/10.1093/jnci/djq229.

Persaud, Nav, Hannah Woods, Aine Workentin, Itunu Adekoya, James R. Dunn, Stephen W. Hwang, Jonathon Maguire, Andrew D. Pinto, Patricia O'Campo, Sean B. Rourke, and Daniel Werb. 2021. "Recommendations for Equitable COVID-19 Pandemic Recovery in Canada." *CMAJ* 193, no. 49 (December): E1878–88. https://doi.org/10.1503/cmaj.210904.

Petersen, Alan. 1997. "Risk, Governance and the New Public Health." In *Foucault: Health and Medicine*, edited by Robin Bunton and Alan Petersen, 189–206. New York: Routledge.

Petryna, Adriana. 2002. *Life Exposed: Biological Citizens after Chernobyl*. Princeton, NJ: Princeton University Press.

Picard, Andre. 2007. "Should HPV Vaccinations Be Extended to Young Men?" *Globe and Mail*, 27 March 2007. https://www.theglobeandmail.com/life /should-hpv-vaccinations-be-extended-to-young-men/article1315154.

– 2008. "HPV and Cancer, Down to a Science." *Globe and Mail*, 21 October 2008. https://www.theglobeandmail.com/technology/science/hpv-and -cancer-down-to-a-science/article1064581.

– 2009. "Teen and Young Adult Cancer Rates Rising." *Globe and Mail*, 16 April 2009. https://www.theglobeandmail.com/incoming/teen-and-young -adult-cancer-rates-rising/article1196253.

– 2010a. "Boys, as Well as Girls, Need HPV Vaccine, Medical Group Says." *Globe and Mail*, 23 November 2010. https://www.theglobeandmail.com/life /health-and-fitness/boys-as-well-as-girls-need-hpv-vaccine-medical-group-says /article559033.

– 2010b. "Doctors Urge HPV Vaccine for Boys." *Globe and Mail*, 24 November 2010.

Poland, Gregory A., and Robert M. Jacobson. 2001. "Understanding Those Who Do Not Understand: A Brief Review of the Anti-vaccine Movement." *Vaccine* 19, no. 17–19 (March): 2440–5. https://doi.org/10.1016 /S0264-410X(00)00469-2.

Poland, Gregory A., Robert M. Jacobson, and Inna G. Ovsyannikova. 2009. "Trends Affecting the Future of Vaccine Development and Delivery: The Role of Demographics, Regulatory Science, the Anti-vaccine Movement, and Vaccinomics." *Vaccine* 27, no. 25–26 (May): 3240–4. https://doi.org /10.1016/j.vaccine.2009.01.069.

Public Health Agency of Canada (PHAC). 2005. *Canadian Human Papillomavirus Vaccine Research Priorities Workshop: Final Report*. Ottawa: PHAC. https://publications.gc.ca/collections/Collection/HP3-3-32S1E.pdf.

Public Health Ontario. 2022. *COVID-19 Vaccine Uptake in Ontario: December 14, 2020 to December 18, 2022*. Toronto: King's Printer for Ontario.

https://www.publichealthontario.ca/-/media/Documents/nCoV/epi
/covid-19-vaccine-uptake-ontario-epi-summary.pdf.

Puxley, Chinta. 2008. "Half of Eligible Grade 8 Girls Declining Free HPV
Vaccine, Ministry Finds." *Globe and Mail,* 18 April 2008. https://www
.theglobeandmail.com/news/national/half-of-eligible-grade-8-girls
-declining-free-hpv-vaccine-ministry-finds/article670980.

Rabin, Roni Caryn. 2009. "Gardasil's "Benefits Still Outweigh the Risks."
Hamilton Spectator, 20 August 2009.

Rapp, Rayna. 1994. "Women's Responses to Prenatal Diagnosis: A Sociocultural
Perspective on Diversity." In *Women and Prenatal Testing: Facing the Challenges
of Genetic Technology,* edited by Karen Rothenberg and Elizabeth Thompson,
219–33. Athens: University of Ohio Press.

– 2007. "Real-Time Fetus: The Role of the Sonogram in the Age of Monitored
Reproduction." In *Beyond the Body Proper: Reading the Anthropology of Material
Life,* edited by Margaret Lock and Judith Farquhar, 608–22. Durham, NC:
Duke University Press.

Reed, Jim. 2021. "Covid Vaccines: Mixing Increases Reports of Mild Side-
Effects." *BBC,* 13 May 2021. https://www.bbc.com/news/health-57075503.

Region of Waterloo. n.d. "HPV." Health and Wellness. Accessed 14 March 2023.
https://www.regionofwaterloo.ca/en/health-and-wellness/hpv.aspx.

Rich, Adrienne. (1976) 1986. *Of Woman Born: Motherhood as Experience and
Institution.* New York: W.W. Norton & Company.

Richens, John, John Imrie, and Helen Weiss. 2003. "Human Immunodeficiency
Risk: Is It Possible to Dissuade People from Having Unsafe Sex?" *Journal of the
Royal Statistical Society: Series A* 166, no. 2 (June): 207–15. https://doi.org
/10.1111/1467-985X.00268.

Roan, Shari. 2007. "Human Papillomavirus from the Male Perspective."
Edmonton Journal, 15 April 2007.

Robbins, Peter. 2008. "A Reckless Decision." Letter to the editor, *Toronto Star,* 6 June
2008. https://www.thestar.com/opinion/2008/06/06/a_reckless_decision.html.

Roche, Brenda, Alan Neaigus, and Maureen Miller. 2005. "Street Smarts
and Urban Myths: Women, Sex Work, and the Role of Storytelling in Risk
Reduction and Rationalization." *Medical Anthropology Quarterly* 19, no. 2
(June): 149–70. https://doi.org/10.1525/maq.2005.19.2.149.

Rosaldo, Michelle. 1974. "Women, Culture, and Society: A Theoretical
Overview." In *Women, Culture, and Society,* edited by Michelle Rosaldo and
Louise Lamphere, 17–42. Stanford, CA: Stanford University Press.

Rose, Nikolas. 2007. *The Politics of Life Itself: Biomedicine, Power, and Subjectivity in
the Twenty-First Century.* Princeton, NJ: Princeton University Press.

Rose, Nikolas, and Carlos Novas. 2005. "Biological Citizenship." In *Global
Assemblages: Technology, Politics, and Ethics as Anthropological Problems,* edited by
S. J. Collier and A. Ong, 439–63. Malden: Blackwell.

Rothstein, Henry. 2006. "The Institutional Origins of Risk: A New Agenda for Risk Research." *Health, Risk & Society* 8 (3): 215–21. https://doi.org /10.1080/13698570600871646.

Russell, Ginny, and Susan Kelly. 2011. "Looking Beyond Risk: A Study of Lay Epidemiology of Childhood Disorders." *Health, Risk & Society* 13 (2): 129–45. https://doi.org/10.1080/13698575.2010.515738.

Saukko, Paula. 2010. "Beyond Pill Scares? Online Discussions on Genetic Thrombophilia and Gendered Contradictions." In *Governing the Female Body: Gender, Health, and Networks of Power*, edited by Lori Reed and Paula Saukko, 40–58. Albany: State University of New York Press.

Sawicki, Jana. 1991. *Disciplining Foucault: Feminism, Power, and the Body*. New York: Routledge. https://doi.org/10.4324/9781003070825.

Scheper-Hughes, Nancy. 1999. "*Nervoso*: Medicine, Sickness, and Human Needs." In *Health Studies: A Critical and Cross-Cultural Reader*, edited by Colin Samson, 338–63. Oxford: Blackwell.

Schneider, Katie. 2012. "Bishop Says Drug Maker Gains Most in HPV Fight." *Calgary Sun*, 30 November 2012.

Scott, Joan W. 1992. "Experience." In *Feminists Theorize the Political*, edited by Judith Butler and Joan W. Scott, 22–40. New York: Routledge. https://doi.org /10.4324/9780203723999.

Shafran, Stephen. 2008. "Fearmongering Is Costing Lives." *National Post*, 23 April 2008.

Sheth, Jagdish N., Rajendra S. Sisodia, and Arun Sharma. 2000. "The Antecedents and Consequences of Customer-Centric Marketing." *Journal of the Academy of Marketing Science* 28, no. 1 (December): 55–66. https://doi.org /10.1177/0092070300281006.

Shoveller, Jean A., Rod Knight, Joy Johnson, John L. Oliffe, and Shira Goldenberg. 2010. "'Not the Swab!' Young Men's Experiences with STI Testing." *Sociology of Health & Illness* 32, no. 1 (January): 57–73. https://doi .org/10.1111/j.1467-9566.2009.01222.x.

Sicoli, Florence. 2009. "Health News." *Hamilton Spectator*, 7 January 2009. https://www.thespec.com/life/2009/01/21/health-news.html.

Silversides, Ann. 2010. "Lifting the Curtain on the Drug Approval Process." In *The Push to Prescribe: Women and Canadian Drug Policy*, edited by Anne Rochon Ford and Diane Saibil, 115–38. Toronto: Women's Press.

Slade, Barbara A., Laura Leidel, Claudia Vellozzi, Emily Jane Woo, Wei Hua, Andrea Sutherland, Hector S. Izurieta, Robert Ball, Nancy Miller, M. Miles Braun, Lauri E. Markowitz, and John Iskander. 2009. "Postlicensure Safety Surveillance for Quadrivalent Human Papillomavirus Recombinant Vaccine." *JAMA* 302, no. 7 (August): 750–7. https://doi.org/10.1001/jama.2009.1201.

Smith-Rosenberg, Carroll. 1989. "The Body Politic." In *Coming to Terms: Feminism, Theory, Politics*, edited by Elizabeth Weed, 101–21. New York: Routledge. https://doi.org/10.4324/9780203093917.

Society of Canadian Colposcopists. 2007. "The Society of Canadian Colposcopists Strongly Endorses the NACI Statement of HPV Vaccination." News release, 22 March 2007.

Society of Gynecologic Oncology of Canada (GOC). 2006. *GOC Position Statement Regarding Prophylactic HPV Vaccines.* Ottawa: GOC.

– 2007. *Gynecologic Oncologists Strongly Endorse NACI Statement of HPV Vaccination.* Toronto: GOC.

– 2012. *GOC Position Statement Regarding NACI Update on Human Papillomavirus (HPV) Vaccines.* Ottawa: GOC.

Society of Obstetricians and Gynaecologists of Canada (SOGC). 2007a. "Canadian Consensus Guidelines on Human Papillomavirus." *Journal of Obstetrics and Gynaecology Canada* 29, no. 8 (August): S1–S60. https://doi.org/10.1016/S1701-2163(16)32573-7.

– 2007b. "SOGC Statement on CMAJ Commentary (August 14), Human Papillomavirus, Vaccines and Women's Health: Questions and Cautions." Accessed 10 October 2012. www.sogc.org/media/guidelines-hpv-commentary_e.asp (site discontinued).

– 2012. "HPV DNA Testing." Accessed 15 November 2012. http:/www.hpvinfo.ca/parents/hpv-dna-testing (site discontinued).

– 2016. "New HPV Campaign Targets Women Ages 25–45." News release, 7 October 2016.

Solomon, Lawrence. 2009. "First, Do No Harm; Those Who Question the Safety of Vaccines Are Being Unfairly Attacked." *National Post,* 23 May 2009.

Sontag, Susan. 1999. "Illness as Metaphor and AIDS and Its Metaphors." In *Health Studies: A Critical and Cross-Cultural Reader,* edited by Colin Samson, 133–49. Oxford: Blackwell.

Spencer, Grace. 2013. "The 'Healthy Self' and 'Risky' Young Other: Young People's Interpretations of Health and Health-Related Risks." *Health, Risk & Society* 15 (5): 449–62. https://doi.org/10.1080/13698575.2013.804037.

Standing Committee on Finance. 2006. FINA Committee Meeting, Number 16, 1st Session, 39th Parliament, 19 September 2006. Ottawa: House of Commons Canada. https://www.ourcommons.ca/DocumentViewer/en/39-1/FINA/meeting-16/evidence.

Standing Committee on the Status of Women. 2005. *Gender-Based Analysis: Building Blocks for Success.* Ottawa: House of Commons. https://publications.gc.ca/collections/collection_2017/parl/xc71-1/XC71-1-1-381-2-eng.pdf.

Status of Women Canada. 1995. *Setting the Stage for the Next Century: The Federal Plan for Gender Equality.* Ottawa: Status of Women Canada. https://publications.gc.ca/collections/Collection/SW21-15-1995E.pdf.

– 2004. *Integrated Approach to Gender-Based Analysis: Information Kit.* Ottawa: Status of Women Canada. http://publications.gc.ca/site/eng/294256/publication.html.

– 2013. "GBA+: Gender-Based Analysis Plus." Accessed 21 May 2013. http://www
.swc-cfc.gc.ca/pol/gba-acs/indexeng.html (site discontinued).

Stewart, Kathleen. 2000. "Real American Dreams (Can Be Nightmares)." In
Cultural Studies and Political Theory, edited by Jodi Dean, 243–57. Ithaca, NY:
Cornell University Press.

– 2005. "Trauma Time: A Still Life." In *Histories of the Future*, edited by Daniel
Rosenberg and Susan Harding, 321–39. Durham, NC: Duke University Press.

Stobbe, Mike. 2011. "Panel Advises HPV Vaccine for Boys." *Globe and Mail*,
26 October 2011.

Streefland, Pieter, A.M.R. Chowdry, and Pilar Ramos-Jimenez. 1999. "Patterns
of Vaccination Acceptance." *Social Science & Medicine* 49, no. 12 (December):
1705–16. https://doi.org/10.1016/S0277-9536(99)00239-7.

Talaga, Tanya. 2007. "Lobbyists Boosted Vaccine Program." *Toronto Star*,
16 August 2007. https://www.thestar.com/news/2007/08/16/lobbyists
_boosted_vaccine_program.html.

Thing, Lone Friis, and Laila Ottesen. 2013. "Young People's Perspectives on
Health, Risks and Physical Activity in a Danish Secondary School." *Health, Risk
& Society* 15 (5): 463–77. https://doi.org/10.1080/13698575.2013.802294.

Thomas, Michelle. 2005. "'What Happens in Tenerife Stays in Tenerife':
Understanding Women's Sexual Behaviour on Holiday." *Culture, Health &
Sexuality* 7 (6): 571–84. https://doi.org/10.1080/13691050500256807.

Thompson, Charis. 2005. *Making Parents: The Ontological Choreography of
Reproductive Technologies*. Cambridge, MA: MIT Press.

– 2007. "Quit Snivelling, Cryo-Baby, We'll Work Out Which One Is Your
Mama." In *Beyond the Body Proper: Reading the Anthropology of Material Life*,
edited by Margaret Lock and Judith Farquhar, 623–39. Durham, NC: Duke
University Press.

Throsby, Karen. 2010. "'Doing What Comes Naturally …' Negotiating
Normality in Accounts of IVF-Failure." In *Governing the Female Body: Gender,
Health, and Networks of Power*, edited by Lori Reed and Paula Saukko, 233–52.
Albany: State University of New York Press.

Thurer, Shari. 1994. *The Myths of Motherhood: How Culture Reinvents the Good
Mother*. Boston: Houghton Mifflin.

Toronto Star. 2015a. "Make Sure Girls and Parents Know Any Risks with the HPV
Vaccine." Editorial, 5 February 2015. https://www.thestar.com/opinion
/editorials/2015/02/05/make-sure-girls-and-parents-know-any-risk-with
-hpv-vaccine-editorial.html.

– 2015b. "A Note from the Publisher." 20 February 2015. https://www.thestar
.com/news/2015/02/20/a-note-from-the-publisher.html.

Trigg, Nicole. 2016. "Editorial: Resistance When Going against the Status Quo."
Invermere Valley Echo, 9 March 2016. https://www.invermerevalleyecho.com
/opinion/editorial-resistance-when-going-against-the-status-quo.

Tsing, Anna. 1993. *In the Realm of the Diamond Queen: Marginality in an Out-of-the-Way Place*. Princeton, NJ: Princeton University Press.

Tudiver, Sari. 2009. "Integrating Women's Health and Gender Analysis in a Government Context: Reflections on a Work in Progress." In *Women's Health: Intersections of Policy, Research and Practice*, edited by Pat Armstrong and Jennifer Deadman, 21–34. Toronto: Women's Press.

Tuinstra, Jolanda, Johan W. Groothoff, Wim J.A. Van Den Heuvel, and Doeke Post. 1998. "Socio-economic Differences in Health Risk Behavior in Adolescence: Do They Exist?" *Social Science & Medicine* 47, no. 1 (July): 67–74. https://doi.org/10.1016/S0277-9536(98)00034-3.

Turner, Bryan. 1997. "From Governmentality to Risk: Some Reflections on Foucault's Contribution to Medical Sociology." In *Foucault: Health and Medicine*, edited by Robin Bunton and Alan Petersen, ix–xxi. New York: Routledge.

Vanslyke, Jan, Julie Baum, Veronica Plaza, Maria Otero, Cosette Wheeler, and Deborah Helitzer. 2008. "HPV and Cervical Cancer Testing and Prevention: Knowledge, Beliefs, and Attitudes among Hispanic Women." *Qualitative Health Research* 18, no. 5 (May): 584–96. https://doi.org/10.1177/1049732308315734.

Victoria Times Colonist. 2008. "Data Shows HPV Vaccine Is Remarkably Safe." 2 September 2008. https://www.timescolonist.com/archive/data-shows-hpv-vaccine-is-remarkably-safe-4589970.

Visweswaran, Kamala. 1994. *Fictions of Feminist Ethnography*. Minneapolis: University of Minnesota Press.

Walls, John, Nick Pidgeon, Andrew Weyman, and Tom Horlick-Jones. 2010. "Critical Trust: Understanding Lay Perceptions of Health and Safety Risk Regulation." *Health, Risk & Society* 6 (2): 133–50. https://doi.org/10.1080/1369857042000219788.

Wardlow, Holly. 2006. *Wayward Women: Sexuality and Agency in a New Guinea Society*. Berkeley: University of California Press.

Wedel, Janine, Cris Shore, Gregory Feldman, and Stacy Lathrop. 2005. "Toward an Anthropology of Public Policy." *AAPSS* 600, no. 1 (July): 30–51. https://doi.org/10.1177/0002716205276734.

Weed, Elizabeth, and Judith Butler. 2011. "Introduction." In *The Question of Gender: Joan W. Scott's Critical Feminism*, edited by Judith Butler and Elizabeth Weed, 1–8. Bloomington: Indiana University Press.

Weeks, Carly. 2012. "Calgary Catholic Schools Finally Lift Ban on HPV Vaccine." *Globe and Mail*, 29 November 2012. https://www.theglobeandmail.com/life/the-hot-button/calgary-catholic-schools-finally-lift-ban-on-hpv-vaccine/article5794968.

– 2014. "Debate over HPV Vaccine Has Nothing to Do with Morality." *Globe and Mail*, 14 December 2014. https://www.theglobeandmail.com/life/health-and-fitness/health/debate-over-hpv-vaccine-has-nothing-to-do-with-morality/article22069521.

Wente, Margaret. 2007. "Prevention Won't Cure Health Care." *Globe and Mail*, 14 August 2007. https://www.theglobeandmail.com/news/national /prevention-wont-cure-health-care/article724858.

Williams, Shoshannah, and Georgina Drew. 2020. "'Co-creating Meeting Spaces': Feminist Ethnographic Fieldwork in Bangladesh." *Gender, Place & Culture* 27 (6): 831–53. https://doi.org/10.1080/0966369X.2019.1657070.

Wilson, Sarah, Emily Karas, Natasha S. Crowcroft, Erika Bontovics, and Shelley L. Deeks. 2012. "Ontario's School-Based HPV Immunization Program: School Board Assent and Parental Consent." *Canadian Journal of Public Health* 103 (1): 34–9. https://doi.org/10.1007/BF03404066.

Wyndham-West, Michelle. 2013. "'What's a Mom to Do?' Negotiating Public Health Literacies through the Traffic between Motherhood and Mothering in School-Based HPV Vaccination Programming." In *Mothering and Literacies*, edited by Amanda B. Richey and Linda Shuford Evans, 274–92. Toronto: Demeter Press.

– 2016. "'It's Really Complicated': Canadian University Women Students Navigate Gendered Risk and Human Papillomavirus (HPV) Vaccine Decision-Making." *Health, Risk & Society* 18 (1–2): 59–76. https://doi.org /10.1080/13698575.2016.1176127.

Wyndham-West, Michelle, Mary Wiktorowicz, and Peter Tsasis. 2017. "Power and Culture in Emerging Medical Technology Policymaking: The Case of the Human Papillomavirus (HPV) Vaccine in Canada." *Evidence & Policy* 14 (2): 277–99. https://doi.org/10.1332/174426417X14845753387144.

Zaloom, Caitlin. 2004. "The Productive Life of Risk." *Cultural Anthropology* 19, no. 3 (January): 365–91. https://doi.org/10.1525/can.2004.19.3.365.

Zechmeister, Ingrid, Birgitte Freiesleben de Blasio, and Geoff Garnett. 2010. "HPV-Vaccination for the Prevention of Cervical Cancer in Austria: A Model Based Long-Term Prognosis of Cancer Epidemiology." *Journal of Public Health* 18 (1): 3–13. https://doi.org/10.1007/s10389-009-0276-3.

Zinn, Jens. 2008. "Heading into the Unknown: Everyday Strategies for Managing Risk and Uncertainty." *Health, Risk & Society* 10 (5): 439–50. https://doi.org/10.1080/13698570802380891.

Zuliani, Janice. 2009. "Versatile Vaccine." *Calgary Herald*, 27 June 2009.

Index

abstinence, 33, 73, 77
access to care, 4, 102, 119
activism, 119
adenovirus vector vaccines, 3
Advisory Committee on
  Immunization Practices (ACIP), 72
agency: and content analysis,
  15; and HPV vaccine decision-
  making, 20, 54, 111, 112, 123n7;
  and HPV vaccine marketing, 83;
  and motherhood, 37; theoretical
  framework, 9–10, 17, 23, 38, 116
Alberta, 67, 74, 96, 106
Allen, Amy, 8, 9, 17, 22, 111, 121n4
allergic reactions, 67. *See also* side
  effects
anthropology, 78, 103
anthropology, medical, 14, 19, 22, 112
anti-archive, 13
anti-science, 72, 75, 79
anti-vaccination, 30–1, 49, 75, 77, 79.
  See also non-acceptance
AstraZeneca, 3, 5
Austria, 109
authentic mothering, 37. *See also*
  mothering and mothers' narratives

barrier protection, 43, 46, 47, 50, 53,
  57. *See also* sexual health

Bartky, Sandra, 89
Beck, Gail, 99
Beck, Ulrich, 121n1, 123n9
Bendixen, Kae, 88
Biehl, João, 14, 90, 122n4
big pharma: mothers on, 27,
  30, 32, 35, 39; university-aged
  women on, 51, 53, 57, 59. *See also*
  pharmaceutical discourses
binaries, 61, 75
biological citizenship, 84. *See also*
  governmentality
biological disruption, 112–13. *See also*
  subjectivities
biomedical approach, 83
birth control, 43, 46, 47, 50, 53, 57.
  See also sexual health
Blackwell, Tom, 78
Blake, Jennifer, 74, 100
blame, 47–8
Blatchford, Andy, 72
blood clots, 5. *See also* side effects
bodies, 33, 56, 66, 84
Boessenkool, Ken, 65, 97
Boholm, Asa, 7, 8, 84, 112, 121n2
born-again Christianity, 34. *See also*
  Christianity
Bourdieu, Pierre, 61
Bourgeault, Ivy, 22

boys. *See* men and boys
Branswell, Helen, 66, 69, 74
breast cancer, 25, 88. *See also* cancer,
　cervical; cancer, HPV related
British Columbia, 96, 97, 106
brochures and pamphlets, 81, 82, 85.
　See also marketing
Brown, Adalsteinn, 118
Brown, Vivian, 99–100
Bury, Michael, 112
Bush, George W., 33, 35
Butler, Judith: on agency, 10, 37,
　38, 55; on gender, 10, 14, 17, 23,
　36, 104; on narratives, 14; on
　self-making, 56, 113; and social
　locations, 105; theory of, 9, 111,
　121n4
Butler-Jons, David, 66

Cairney, Paul, 61
Calgary Herald, 64, 67–8, 71
Canada AM, 72
*Canadian Consensus Guidelines on
　Human Papillomavirus*, 99
*Canadian Human Papillomavirus Vaccine
　Research Priorities Workshop*, 93
Canadian Immunization Committee
　(CIC), 95–6, 101
Canadian Medical Association, 73
*Canadian Medical Association Journal
　(CMAJ)*, 64–5, 94–5
Canadian Paediatric Society, 62, 70
Canadian Pharmacists Association, 62
Canadian Press, 68, 72, 73
cancer, 88–9, 122n6
cancer, cervical: future
　considerations, 119; and GBA,
　101–2; and HPV vaccine decision-
　making, 35, 39; and HPV vaccine
　marketing, 26, 30, 52, 82, 89–91;
　and HPV vaccine policymaking, 25,
　92, 93, 94, 95; media coverage on,

60, 62, 63–5, 67, 68, 69, 70, 73, 74,
　78; and risk, theories of, 88
cancer, HPV related: future
　considerations, 109; gendering
　of, 6, 10, 93, 101; and HPV
　strains, 123n1; and HPV vaccine
　marketing, 18, 52, 80, 81, 86, 89–
　91; and HPV vaccine policymaking,
　92, 93, 95; media coverage on,
　63–5, 69, 70–1, 72, 73, 74. *See also*
　cancer, cervical
Cancer Care Ontario, 63, 122n6
categorical-content analysis, 14–15.
　See also methodology
Catholicism, 67, 73–4, 77
Catholic schools, 34, 68–9, 70–1,
　73–4, 75
Cervarix, 93. *See also* Gardasil
cervical cancer. *See* cancer, cervical;
　cancer, HPV related
choreography, ontological,
　112–13. *See also* ontological
　decision-making
Chowdry, A.M.R., 54
Christianity, 21, 34–5, 75. *See also*
　Catholicism
citizenship, biological, 84. *See also*
　governmentality
City of Toronto, 21, 73, 95
class, category of, 121–2n6, 124n1
clinics, 6, 12, 50, 73, 85, 111
coding, 15. *See also* methodology
coercion, 49. *See also* HPV vaccine
　decision-making
College of Family Physicians of
　Canada, 99
commercials, 81, 82, 85. *See also*
　marketing
communication, 4, 45–6, 55–6, 58,
　69. *See also* negotiation, health
condoms, 43, 46, 47, 50, 53, 57.
　See also sexual health

Condyloma acuminata (genital warts), 41, 42–5, 57, 68, 69, 86, 89
connected critics, 22
Connel, Erin, 84
consumerism, 82, 83, 84. *See also* marketing
contaminants, 31. *See also* HPV vaccine decision-making
content analysis, 14–15. *See also* methodology
continuity of care, 42–3
contraceptives, 43, 46, 47, 50, 53, 57. *See also* sexual health
Cormier, Renée, 105, 119
cost-benefit analysis, 114–15. *See also* decision-making
cost-effectiveness, 101–2. *See also* gender-based analysis
Cotter, John, 96
Couric, Katie, 68
COVID-19, 3–5
Crenshaw, Kimberlé, 105
Crighton, E.J., 114–15
critical discourse analysis, 61. *See also* methodology

Das, Veena, 56
data, 14–15, 111. *See also* information, health; methodology
Dean, Mitchell, 8, 83
"Debate Begins over Public Funding for HPV Vaccine" (Comeau), 94–5
de Beauvoir, Simone, 89
decision-making, 4–5, 8, 9, 114–15. *See also* HPV vaccine decision-making; ontological decision-making
de-gendering, 54–6, 59, 71–2, 73, 74, 79, 99–100, 115. *See also* gender and gendering discourses
Del Grande, Michael, 75
depression, 43

deviance, 7, 48, 56, 61, 78. *See also* promiscuity
direct-to-consumer advertising, 83, 84. *See also* marketing
disability, 3, 21, 56, 104
disease specificity, 117, 118
diversity analysis, 102–3. *See also* gender-based analysis
doctors. *See* medical professionals
"Does Vaccine Turn Girls into Guinea Pigs?" (Henry), 67–8
doing, act of: and mothering, 22–3, 36, 38, 39–40, 113–14, 116–17; theoretical framework, 17; and university-aged women, 54, 55, 56, 114, 116–17
doses, 3, 4–5, 25, 69, 74, 96, 106, 108
Douglas, Mary, 9, 13, 86–7, 89, 101, 105, 111, 121n4
dysplasia, cervical, 29, 41, 44, 52, 57, 59, 112

Edmonton Journal, 64, 69–70, 71
education, sexual health, 16, 41, 44, 46–7, 55–6, 58, 59, 122n7. *See also* sexual health
education rates, 122n2
efficacy, 64, 66, 67, 71, 73, 79
egg (reproductive cell), 88
Elwood, Liz, 63
empowerment, 47, 48, 55, 81. *See also* subjectivities
English, Kathy, 76–7
epidemiology, 83, 109
Epstein, Steven, 35
equity, 3, 4, 6, 73, 96, 97, 118–19
eradication, 68
ethical subjects. *See* agency; subjectivities
ethnographic fieldwork, 10, 14, 19, 22, 110, 121n5
etiology, 118

Ewald, Francois, 7
experiences: and class, category of, 121–2n6; definitions and theory, 13–14, 112; of HPV infection, 41, 42–5; and HPV vaccine decision-making, 15, 20, 22, 27, 29, 35, 37–8, 39, 52, 53–4, 57–9; and narratives or interviews, 19, 21–2; and ontological decision-making, 114–15
expert knowledge, 82. *See also* Foucault, Michel; knowledge formation

Factiva, 60–1. *See also* information, health
faith and religion. *See* Catholicism; Catholic schools
Farquhar, Judith, 22
fear: and HPV vaccine decision-making, 26, 32, 38, 43; and media coverage, 26, 63, 74, 76; and sales/governance strategies, 18, 32, 38, 80, 83, 90–1; and STIs, 56
federal government: and GBA, 19, 92, 100, 101–2, 104, 105; and HPV vaccine, 21, 32, 93–4, 95, 124n2; and HPV vaccine policymaking, 11, 18, 92, 97–8, 100, 109, 110; media coverage of, 62, 65; sales/governance strategies of, 115–16; and transparency, 117. *See also* governmental discourses
Federal Plan for Gender Equality, The, 100, 102–3
Federation of Medical Women of Canada (FMWC), 71–2, 99, 100
feminist theory, 8–9, 13, 17, 103–4, 121n4
fidelity, 45, 55, 58
fieldwork, ethnographic, 10, 14, 19, 22, 110, 121n5
"First, Do No Harm; Those Who Question the Safety of Vaccines

Are Being Unfairly Attacked" (Solomon), 71
fluidity, 117, 118. *See also* gender and gendering discourses
flu shot, 26, 31
Food and Drug Administration (FDA), 71, 82; and COVID-19, 3
Forth World Conference on Women, 100
Foucault, Michel: on governmentality, 9, 83; on knowledge, 82; masculine pronouns, usage of, 121n4; on power, 78, 83, 87, 89, 90, 111; and risk, theories of, 11; on subjectivity, 9–10, 17, 23, 37, 122n8; on surveillance, 89; on truths, 61
Fox, Nick, 7

Gardasil: approval of, 93, 94, 95, 123n4; governmental discourses on, 25, 82, 84, 85; marketing of, 6, 11, 12, 26–7, 32, 47, 81, 82–3, 84, 85, 89; media coverage of, 65, 66, 68, 69, 71, 76, 77; university-aged women on, 50, 51
Gardasil-9, 96
gender and gendering discourses: and COVID-19 vaccines, 4–5; and GBA, 100–5, 117, 118–19; and HPV vaccine, 6; and HPV vaccine decision-making, 47–9, 51, 57, 110, 111, 112–13; and HPV vaccine marketing, 47–8, 80–3, 84, 85–6, 89–91, 103, 110; and HPV vaccine policymaking, 10–11, 92, 93–7, 99–100, 105, 109, 116; interviews on, 12–13, 15; and media coverage, 62, 63, 64, 66, 68, 69, 70, 71–2, 74; and mothers' narratives, 16, 22, 27, 36, 39, 111; reordering of, 19, 113–14, 116–17; research questions, 9, 10, 12, 110; and risk, theories of, 8–9,

10, 11, 84, 86–90, 109, 110; and
sales/governance strategies, 10–11,
18–19; theoretical framework,
10, 13, 17–18, 20, 23, 104; and
university-aged women, 16, 41,
47–9, 53, 54–5, 56, 58–9
gender-based analysis (GBA), 19, 92,
100–4, 109, 110, 117, 118
gender-based analysis plus (GBA+),
4, 11, 13, 18–19, 92, 105, 118–19
generative pause, 17, 20, 22–3, 112,
116–17. *See also* subjectivities
genitalia, 88–9. *See also* sex and sexuality
genital warts, 41, 42–5, 57, 68, 69,
86, 89
Giddens, Anthony, 16–17, 57, 84
Ginn, Diana, 37
Giroux, Henry, 83, 84, 124n3
GlaxoSmithKline Biologicals, 93. *See
also* pharmaceutical discourses
Glenn, Evelyn N., 37
Globe and Mail: HPV vaccine, negative
coverage of, 67; HPV vaccine
endorsement, 63, 64, 68–9, 70, 71,
72, 73, 75; medical societies in,
62–3, 66; neutral coverage, 74; and
"What's the hurry?" narrative, 64–5
Goffman, Irving, 16, 56
Gold, Ronald, 77
Good, Byron, 14, 122n4
good mothers: and HPV vaccine
decision-making, 22, 32, 35, 37, 38,
39–40, 113, 117; and HPV vaccine
marketing, 26–7, 36, 85, 103; and
ontological decision-making, 20,
114, 115. *See also* mothering and
mothers' narratives
governance strategies. *See* sales/
governance strategies
governmental discourses: and GBA,
13, 19, 92, 100, 101–2, 104, 105;
and HPV vaccine, 6, 13, 19, 20, 21,

32, 60, 93–4, 95; and HPV vaccine
decision-making, 16, 17, 18,
24–5, 34, 47–8, 116, 117; and HPV
vaccine marketing, 84, 87, 91, 103;
and HPV vaccine policymaking, 11,
12, 18, 65–6, 84, 92, 95, 97–8, 104,
109, 115–16; and media coverage,
62, 63, 65, 70, 71; and mothers'
narratives, 22, 24–5, 27, 35–6, 37,
39; theoretical framework, 13; and
university-aged women, 16, 41, 46,
47, 49–51, 52, 54, 56
governmentality, 9, 61, 83–4, 111,
121n1, 121n3
Graham, Janice, 93–4
grand theory, 7, 112. *See also* situated
risk
grants, 70, 98–9
Gregg, Jessica, 54
Grier, Jason, 65, 98
Guelph Mercury, 63
Guichon, Juliet, 76
Gulli, Cathy, 60, 65–6
gynaecology, 88–9

H1N1 vaccine, 31, 32
Ha, Tu Thanh, 67
Halton Catholic District School Board,
34, 68–9. *See also* Catholic schools
Hamilton Spectator, 63, 71
Hankivsky, Olena, 11, 100, 101, 102,
105, 119
Hanson, Barbara, 88–9
Harper, Diane M., 67
Hayes, Sharon, 36
Health Canada, 3, 72, 93–4, 95–6,
97–8, 100–1, 122n1
healthism, 7. *See also* self-regulation
Health Sector Payment Transparency
Act (2017), 117–18
health strategies, 36, 38. *See also*
doing, act of

Henry, Fred, 67–8, 74
hepatitis B vaccine, 6
herpes, 43. *See also* sexually
transmitted infections
Hill+Knowlton, 65, 97, 98
historicizing, 13–14
HIV, 73, 106, 108, 109
H. Krueger and Associates, 102
Hobson-West, Tru, 115
Holzer, Boris, 123n9
homelessness, 119
HPV infection: and cancer, 123n1;
gendering of, 6, 17, 25, 64, 80,
93, 97, 101, 109, 116; and HPV
vaccine decision-making, 15, 29,
35, 52, 53–4, 58–9; media coverage
on, 63–4, 69; and motherhood,
22; and policymaking, future,
118; research questions, 10;
strains, 123n6; and subjectivities,
17; transmission, 123nn2–3; and
university-aged women, 12, 16, 41,
42–6, 56–7, 58
HPVinfo.ca, 85–6
HPV vaccine: approval of, 93, 94,
95, 123n4; development of, 6;
future considerations, 117, 118–19;
research questions, 9, 10, 12;
uptake rates, 60, 64, 69, 71, 74.
See also Gardasil; HPV vaccine
decision-making; sales/governance
strategies
HPV vaccine decision-making:
interviews on, 12–13, 14, 17; and
media coverage, 18, 60, 66, 70,
74, 76, 79; of mothers, 21–40;
overview, 6–7, 15–16, 111; research
questions, 9, 12, 110; theoretical
framework, 9, 15, 17–18, 19, 20,
112, 113–14; and transparency,
117; of university-aged women,
41–59

"HPV Vaccine Prevents Genital
Lesions in Men, Merck Study
Claims" (Cowan), 68
"HPV – You Could Be at Risk"
(YouTube video), 86. *See also*
information, health
Huff, April N., 35
Hughes, Rachel, 13
husbands, 29–30, 32

Indigenous peoples, 104, 105, 109,
119
individual-as-enterprise, 7. *See also*
self-regulation
individualization, 8, 54, 59, 115, 116
infants, 30–1, 63
information, health: and COVID-19,
4–5; and HPV vaccine, 11, 18,
24–5; and HPV vaccine decision-
making, 24, 48, 50, 51, 52, 60; and
HPV vaccine marketing, 26–7, 82,
85–6; media coverage on, 26, 60–1,
67, 69, 74, 76–7; and transparency,
117–18
intensity, 17, 22. *See also*
intersubjective space
intensive mothering, 36–7, 38, 115.
See also mothering and mothers'
narratives
intersectionality, 14, 92, 102–4, 105,
109, 119
intersubjective space, 9, 14, 17, 22–3,
37, 40, 111, 122n4
interviews: methodology, 11–13, 19,
21–2; participants, 21, 24, 41–2,
122n9; and subjectivities, 14–15,
17, 22–3, 111, 116
Invermere Valley Echo, 77–8

Johnson & Johnson, 3
Journal of American Medical Association
(JAMA), 71

Journal of Obstetrics and Gynaecology Canada, 99

Katie Couric Show, 68
Kaufert, Patricia, 121n2
Kaul, Rupert, 76
Kleinman, Arthur, 14, 122n4
knowledge formation, 11, 20, 21, 61, 82, 89
Kubacki, Maria, 62

Labrador, 107
lactating women, 5
Lawrence, Susan, 88
Lear, Dana, 122n7
legislation, 12, 84, 102, 117–18. *See also* policy and policymaking
Leung, Wendy, 74
Lexchin, Joel, 94
LGBTQ2+ community, 42, 104, 105, 122n3. *See also* men who have sex with men
Lieber, Eugene, 71
Lieblich, Amia, 14–15
Lippman, Abby, 64–5
living (conceptual frame), 22, 23. *See also* intersubjective space
lobbying: and HPV, gendering of, 71–2, 82; and HPV vaccine, 19, 60–1, 110–11; and HPV vaccine decision-making, 32; and HPV vaccine policymaking, 92, 97–9, 109; and media coverage, 65, 78, 79; registration of, 117–18
Lock, Margaret, 22, 121n2
long COVID, 3, 4
loop electrosurgical excision procedures (LEEP), 44, 52
Lopinski, Bob, 65, 98
low-tech interventions, 4
Lupton, Deborah, 121n4; on new public health, 84; on risk, 7, 8,

9, 20, 83, 121n3; on women and medicine, 87, 89, 111

MacDonald, Margaret, 22
Maclean's, 60, 65–6, 68
Mah, Catherine L., 60, 64
Mallick, Heather, 76
Manitoba, 106
Mansi, James, 69–70, 71
manufactured uncertainty, 121n1. *See also* risk; uncertainty
Marcus, George E., 14
marginalized populations, 64, 102, 103, 109, 118
marketing: and desexualization, 35; and HPV vaccine decision-making, 18; and HPV vaccine policymaking, 80–1, 84, 90, 97; of Merck Frosst, 6, 11, 12, 26–7, 41, 64, 80–1, 84, 103, 109–11; and mothering, 16, 32, 38, 81, 82–3, 85–6, 103; and risk, 80, 82, 84, 87, 89–91; of SOGC, 19, 84–6; and university-aged women, 12, 16, 47–8, 49, 50, 51–2
Martin, Emily, 88
McGuinty, Dalton, 65, 68, 95
media coverage of COVID-19, 4–5
media coverage of HPV vaccine: and anti-science narrative, 72, 75, 79; and decision-making, 16, 18, 25–6, 37, 52, 70; and HPV infection, 6; and marketing, 91; negative, 65–6, 67–8, 71, 73–4, 77; neutral, 66, 67, 71, 74; overview, 11, 18, 60–2, 70, 111; and policymaking, 78–9, 93, 97, 116; positive or endorsing, 62–4, 67, 68–73, 74–5, 77, 78; *Toronto Star* vs. public health, 75–7; *Vaccine* journal controversy, 77–8; "What's the hurry?" narrative, 60, 62, 64–5
medical professionals: and HPV infection, 42–3; and HPV vaccine

medical professionals (*continued*)
decision-making, 27, 28, 29, 35, 39;
and media coverage, 61, 62, 65,
67, 69, 70, 71, 72, 73, 75, 77; and
sales/governance strategies, 12, 26,
50, 78, 82, 83, 93, 95
medical societies: and HPV vaccine
marketing, 80–1, 84–6, 91; and
HPV vaccine policymaking, 92; and
lobbying, 19, 61, 98–9; and media
coverage, 18, 62–3, 65, 70–2, 73,
74, 78; on school-based programs,
11; and transparency, 117–18. *See
also* Society of Obstetricians and
Gynaecologists of Canada
medicine, history of, 87–9
men and boys: and Gardasil
approval, 123n4; and GBA, 101–2;
and HPV vaccine marketing, 49,
80–1, 85, 89, 90; and HPV vaccine
policymaking, 92, 94–7, 99–100;
media coverage on, 64, 68, 70, 71–
2, 74; and medicine, history of, 88,
89; in school-based programs, 10,
11, 19, 106–8; and sexual health
negotiation, 55, 56; and STIs, 47,
48, 59; and subjectivities, 17
men who have sex with men (MSM),
96, 106–8, 109, 119. *See also*
LGBTQ2+ community
Merck Frosst: author's experience
with, 122n7; FDA application, 71;
and HPV vaccine policymaking, 60,
92, 93, 94, 109; lobbying of, 19, 61,
97–9, 109; marketing, gender-based,
6, 11, 12, 26–7, 41, 64, 80–1, 84, 103,
109–11; and media coverage, 61,
64, 65, 68, 69–70, 74, 78; and neo-
liberalism, 124n3; sales/governance
strategies of, 11, 78, 82–3, 85, 89–91,
115–16; and transparency, 118

"Merck-Sponsored Study Suggests
HPV Vaccine Benefits Men Too"
(Fox), 68
methodology, 10–15, 21–2, 60–1,
110–11
Moderna, 3, 5
monogamy, 45, 55
Montreal Gazette, 63, 74
Moore, Sarah, 8, 9, 10, 11, 20, 54,
112, 121n4
morality, 34–5, 48, 54, 73, 75, 83, 86–7
mortality rates, 25, 102
mothering and mothers' narratives:
and adolescent sexuality, 33–5; and
governmental discourses, 22, 24–5,
35–6, 37, 39; and HPV vaccine
decision-making, 18, 20, 22, 24–5,
26–33, 35–6, 37–40, 112–14, 116–
17; and HPV vaccine marketing,
16, 32, 38, 81, 82–3, 85–6, 103;
and media coverage, 25–6; and
ontological decision-making, 114–
15; overview, 15–16, 21–2, 24, 111;
and pharmaceutical discourses,
22, 26–7, 30, 32, 35, 37, 38, 39; and
religion, 34–5; and sexual health,
29; theoretical framework, 22–3,
36–8, 40, 112, 116; university-aged
women, compared, 55
mRNA vaccines, 3
Murphy, Joan, 70

narratives, 9, 14–15, 17, 19, 22. *See
also* interviews
National Advisory Committee on
Immunization (NACI), 5, 63, 70,
94, 95–6, 99–100
National Post, 63–4, 68, 70, 71, 78
Native Women's Association of
Canada (NWAC), 104
Naus, Monika, 69

negative agency, 123n7. *See also* non-acceptance

negotiation, health: and ontological decision-making, 20, 111, 114; of university-aged women, 16, 41, 45–7, 53, 55–6, 57, 58, 59

neo-liberalism, 7, 56, 59, 83, 84, 115, 124n3

Nettleton, Sarah, 9, 23, 83, 111, 121n4

New Brunswick, 107

Newfoundland, 96–7, 107

new public health, 7, 10, 23, 56, 83, 84, 115–16. *See also* public health

Nobel Prize, 6, 69

non-acceptance: of mothers, 30–3, 38, 113–14; as reordering, 117; and risk, 123n7; and subpolitics, 123n9; of university-aged women, 16, 41, 49–50, 53, 54–5, 57, 115

Northwest Territories, 107

Novas, Carlos, 84

Nova Scotia, 96, 107

Nunavut, 107

Office of the Commissioner of Lobbying of Canada, 97. *See also* lobbying

Office of the Integrity Commissioner, 98. *See also* transparency

Omicron (COVID-19 variant), 3–4, 5

Ontario, 3, 25, 34, 95–8, 107, 109, 117–18

ontological choreography, 112–13

ontological decision-making, 15, 19, 20, 112–15. *See also* HPV vaccine decision-making

oral sex, 72. *See also* sex and sexuality

O'Reilly, Andrea, 37

Ortner, Sherry, 103

Ottawa Citizen, 62, 64

"Our Girls Are Not Guinea Pigs" (Gulli), 60, 65–6, 68

ova, 88

over-medicalization, 50

Page, Shelley, 65

pandemics, 3–5

Pandolfi, Mariella, 17, 22–3

Paoletti, Jo B., 99

Pap tests: access to, 102, 119; and HPV vaccine decision-making, 28, 29, 30, 44, 50, 52, 57; and media coverage, 64–5

parenting, 46. *See also* mothering and mothers' narratives

patriarchy, 36

pause, generative, 17, 20, 22–3, 112, 116–17. *See also* subjectivities

Pellizzari, Rosana, 73

Petersen, Alan, 7, 84

Petryna, Adriana, 104

Pfizer, 3, 5

pharmaceutical discourses: desexualization in, 35; and HPV vaccine, 6, 19, 60–1, 110–11; and HPV vaccine decision-making, 17, 18, 30, 32, 35, 36, 117; and HPV vaccine marketing, 26, 82, 83, 84, 87, 90–1, 103, 104–5; and HPV vaccine policymaking, 92, 93, 115–16; and media coverage, 65, 71, 77–9; and mothers' narratives, 22, 26–7, 30, 32, 35, 37, 38, 39; research questions, 10; and smart regulation, 94; theoretical framework, 13; and transparency, 117–18; and university-aged women, 41, 47–8, 49, 50–4, 57

Pharmaceutical Drugs Directorate, 94

Pharmaceutical Executive (magazine), 81

physicians. *See* medical professionals
Picard, Andre, 69, 71
policy and policymaking: definitions,
12; future considerations, 117–19;
and GBA, 100–4, 105, 109; and
HPV vaccine, 6, 11, 12, 19, 60,
92–7, 110; and HPV vaccine
marketing, 80–1, 84, 90, 97; and
lobbying, 97–9; research questions,
9, 10; and sales/governance
strategies, 84, 115–16; and
subjectivities, 104–5. *See also* sales/
governance strategies
positionalities, 14, 21–2, 105
power: and GBA+, 105; and HPV
vaccine decision-making, 111,
113–14, 117, 121n2; and HPV
vaccine marketing, 80, 83, 90;
and interview strategies, 13; and
motherhood, 37; and risk, theories
of, 87; and sales/governance
strategies, 9, 18, 61, 78, 82; and
sex/sexuality, 89; and sexual
health negotiation, 47, 55, 56; and
subjectivities, 10, 17, 23
practices of the self, 9, 17, 23. *See also*
subjectivities
pregnancy, 5, 43, 51
pre-marital sex, 34, 69. *See also* sex
and sexuality
"Premier Scolds Board for Refusing
HPV Vaccine" (Canadian Press),
68
prepatients, 84. *See also* governance
strategies
prevention, 7–8, 28, 29, 47, 66, 83–4.
See also Pap tests; screening
Prince Edward Island, 74, 96, 107
privatization of risk, 7. *See also* risk
promiscuity, 32, 34, 48, 73. *See also*
deviance
pronouns, 121n4

provincial governments: and
COVID-19, 4; and HPV vaccine
decision-making, 24–5, 34, 47–8,
116; and media coverage, 62, 70;
and policymaking, 11, 12, 18,
65–6, 84, 92, 95, 97–8, 109; and
public health, 124n2; school-based
programs of, 10, 21, 66, 72, 74,
100, 105. *See also specific provinces*
psycho-socioenvironmental
approach, 83
puberty, 33
public health: and COVID-19, 3, 4;
and HPV, gendering of, 80, 82; and
HPV vaccine, 6, 60, 62; and HPV
vaccine decision-making, 24–5; and
HPV vaccine policymaking, 92; and
media coverage, 18, 64, 66, 73, 75–
7; research questions, 9; and risk,
theories of, 7; and sex education,
56. *See also* governmental
discourses
Public Health Agency of Canada
(PHAC), 60, 64, 66, 69, 76, 93,
101–2

Quebec, 108

Ramos-Jimenez, Pilar, 54
Rapp, Rayna, 124n1
rationality vs. irrationality, 75, 79
Regroupement des Gynécologues
Oncologues du Québec (RGOQ),
70
regulation, smart, 93–4. *See also* policy
and policymaking
reordering, 17, 19, 20, 37, 39, 56,
112–14, 116–17. *See also* HPV
vaccine decision-making
reproduction, 36, 53, 82, 88
research questions, 9, 10, 12, 13,
110–11

resistance, 16, 31, 38, 54, 55, 56, 60.
   See also non-acceptance
"Resistance When Going against the
   Status Quo" (Trigg), 77–8
responsibility, 26, 29, 41, 51, 53, 83,
   84, 98
Rich, Adrienne, 36
risk: and COVID-19, 4–5; and
   GBA, 102; and gender, 8–9, 10,
   11, 84, 86–90, 109, 110; and
   governmentality, 83–4, 111; and
   HPV vaccine decision-making, 6–7,
   12–13, 15–16, 110, 111, 112–13;
   and HPV vaccine marketing,
   80, 82, 84, 87, 89–91; and HPV
   vaccine policymaking, 92, 96,
   110, 116; media coverage of, 62,
   65–6, 67–8, 70–1, 74, 75–7, 78;
   and mothers' narratives, 22, 24,
   28–9, 31–2, 35, 38–9, 111; and
   ontological decision-making, 114–
   15; and policymaking, 104–5; and
   reordering, 19, 113–14, 116–17;
   research questions, 9, 10, 12; and
   sales/governance strategies, 7–8,
   18–19, 83–4, 112, 121n1; and
   sexual health negotiation, 45;
   situated, 7–8, 19–20, 59, 84, 112,
   114–15, 117, 121n2; theoretical
   framework, 7–9, 11, 13, 17–18,
   20, 57; and trust, 16–17; and
   university-aged women, 41, 48–51,
   52, 53, 55, 56–7, 58, 59; and youth,
   123n8
Rosaldo, Michelle, 103
Rose, Nikolas, 84
Rothstein, Henry, 84

sales/governance strategies: and
   COVID-19, 4; and HPV vaccine,
   11, 18, 110–11, 115–16; and HPV
   vaccine decision-making, 18;

and HPV vaccine marketing, 80,
   82–3, 89–91, 115–16; and media
   coverage, 78–9; and policy, 84,
   115–16; reordering of, 19, 20,
   54, 56, 114, 116; and research
   methods, 13; and risk, theories of,
   7–8, 18–19, 83–4, 112, 121n1; of
   SOGC, 84–6; and transparency,
   117; and university-aged women,
   54, 58. *See also* governmental
   discourses; pharmaceutical
   discourses
Saskatchewan, 108
Sawicki, Jana, 13
school-based programs: in Canada,
   105–8; and HPV vaccine
   marketing, 6, 80, 81, 84, 85–6, 90;
   and HPV vaccine policymaking,
   10, 18, 19, 92, 95–7, 100, 116; and
   lobbying, 11, 98; media coverage
   on, 25–6, 64, 68–9, 70, 72, 73–5,
   78; and mothers' narratives, 12,
   16, 21, 24, 32, 34, 35–6, 39, 111;
   university-aged women on, 16, 41,
   46, 47–8, 55–6, 58
"Science Shows HPV Vaccine Has
   No Dark Side" (Guichon and
   Kaul), 76
scientific mothers, 36. *See also*
   mothering and mothers' narratives
Scott, Joan, 13, 14, 121–2n6
screening, 47, 88–9. *See also* Pap tests;
   prevention
secularization, 75
security, 17, 57. *See also* trust
segmented marketing, 81. *See also*
   marketing
self-mastery, 15. *See also* agency
self-reflexivity, 9, 17, 23. *See also*
   subjectivities
self-regulation, 7, 10, 23, 82, 83–4, 116.
   See also sales/governance strategies

sex (biological category), 8, 61, 89
sex and sexuality: and marketing,
 89–90; media coverage on, 69, 72,
 75; mothers on adolescent, 32–5,
 38–9; and risk, 88–9; and STIs, 43,
 48, 53; university-aged women on,
 16, 44–7, 50, 51, 55–6, 57, 58
sexual health: education, 16, 41,
 44, 46–7, 55–6, 58, 59, 122n7;
 gendering of, 51, 53; and HPV
 vaccine decision-making, 28, 29,
 59; and HPV vaccine marketing,
 81; and media coverage, 69, 72,
 73–4, 75; negotiation of, 45–7,
 55–6, 57, 58; and STIs, 43, 58
sexually transmitted infections
 (STIs): gendering of, 47–8,
 53; and HPV vaccine decision-
 making, 52; and HPV vaccine
 marketing, 89, 90; and sales/
 governance strategies, 18, 80; and
 sex education, 56; university-aged
 women on, 16, 41, 42–5, 47–8, 50,
 56, 58–9; and women, 88
Shapiro, Marla, 72
Sharma, Arun, 81
Sheth, Jagdish N., 81
Shoveller, Jean A., 15
side effects: and COVID-19 vaccines,
 4–5; of HPV vaccine, 5; media
 coverage on, 65, 67, 69–70, 75–7;
 mothers' narratives on, 24, 25, 32,
 39; university-aged women on, 41,
 49–50, 52, 57, 58, 59
Sisodia, Rajendra S., 81
situated gender, 8, 19–20, 112, 114–
 15, 117, 121n2. See also gender and
 gendering discourses
situated risk, 7–8, 19–20, 59, 84, 112,
 114–15, 117, 121n2. See also risk
smallpox vaccine, 54

smart regulation, 93–4. See also policy
 and policymaking
Smitherman, George, 65
Smith-Rosenberg, Carroll, 14
Society of Canadian Colposcopists
 (SCC), 70, 99
Society of Gynecologic Oncology of
 Canada (GOC), 62–3, 70, 99, 100
Society of Obstetricians and
 Gynaecologists of Canada (SOGC):
 and HPV vaccine marketing,
 10–11, 19, 80, 84–6, 90, 97; and
 HPV vaccine policymaking, 100;
 and lobbying, 98–9; and media
 coverage, 62, 65, 70, 74
Solomon, Lawrence, 71
S'rensen, Mads P., 123n9
sperm, 88
Status of Women Canada, 105
stereotypes, 6, 59, 61, 66, 73
Stewart, Kathleen, 17, 22
stigma: and HPV infection, 15, 43,
 53, 58, 59, 114; and HPV vaccine,
 32; and sexual education, 16; and
 STIs, 41, 47, 54, 56
still life, 17, 22. See also subjectivities
STIs. See sexually transmitted
 infections
Stobbe, Mike, 72
Streefland, Pieter, 54
stress, 24, 27, 30, 32, 35, 39. See also
 HPV vaccine decision-making
subjectivities: and experiences,
 13, 14; and HPV vaccine
 decision-making, 9–10, 16–20,
 54, 111, 112, 113–14, 117; and
 HPV vaccine marketing, 83;
 and intersectionality, 105; and
 mothering, 22–3, 36, 37, 39, 122n8;
 and narratives, 14, 17, 116; and
 neo-liberalism, 124n3; and policy,

104–5; and university-aged women, 55, 56, 57, 59
subordination, 51, 87–8, 103–4
subpolitics, 123n9
Summary Basis of Decision, 94, 95
surveillance, 10, 83–4, 88–9
Sweet, Lamont, 96
symptoms, 44, 47, 48, 86, 123n2

Talaga, Tanya, 65, 98
technology, emerging, 4, 6, 17, 57, 59, 70, 73–4
telos, 9–10, 17, 23, 56, 57, 111. *See also* subjectivities
textbooks, medical, 88
theoretical framework, 6–10, 17–18
Therapeutic Products Directorate, 94
thesis of book, 19
Thompson, Charis, 112
Thompson, E.P., 121–2n6
Thurer, Shari, 36
Toronto, City of, 21, 73, 95
Toronto Public Health, 95
Toronto Star, 18, 60, 65, 69, 70, 75–7, 98
transcriptions, 15
transmission, 8, 45, 71, 89, 95, 99, 118, 123nn2–3
transparency, 76–7, 98, 117–18
treatment, 44, 57, 63, 66, 83
Trigg, Nicole, 77–8
trust, 4, 15–17, 45, 51, 57–8. *See also* HPV vaccine decision-making
truths, 61, 78
Tsasis, Peter, 98
Tuval-Mashiach, Rivka, 14–15

uncertainty: and COVID-19, 4; and HPV vaccine decision-making, 15–17, 35, 39, 41, 50, 52, 57, 59; manufactured, 121n1; and trust, 16–17, 57

underserviced populations, 19, 118. *See also* marginalized populations
unfreedom, 23. *See also* agency
United Nations, 104
university-aged women: HPV experiences of, 42–4; and HPV vaccine decision-making, 16, 20, 41, 47–59, 112–14, 116–17; and HPV vaccine marketing, 12, 16, 49, 50, 51–2, 81, 85; and ontological decision-making, 114–15; overview, 41–2, 111; on sex education, 33–4, 41, 46–7, 55–6, 58; and sexual health negotiation, 45–7; subjectivities of, 55, 56, 57, 59

Vaccine (journal), 75, 77–8
"Vaccine Could End Most Cervical Cancer: Study; HPV Shots Urged for Older Women" (Blackwell), 68
"Vaccine Debate Is One We Shouldn't Even Be Having" (Mallick), 76
vaccine hesitancy, 4. *See also* non-acceptance; uncertainty
vaccine-induced immune thrombotic thrombocytopenia (VITT), 3. *See also* side effects
Vancouver Sun, 62, 65
Victoria Times Colonist, 67
virginity, 45, 48, 54, 123n3. *See also* sex and sexuality
Visweswaran, Kamala, 103, 105, 109
vulnerability and vulnerable populations: and COVID-19, 4, 5; and decision-making, 20, 29, 115; and HPV vaccine, 6, 11, 41, 66, 92, 106, 108, 119; and risk, theories of, 20; and sexual health, 45, 46–7, 53–4, 55, 56, 58–9, 114. *See also* risk

Walls, John, 58
Wardlow, Holly, 123n7
Waterloo Region Record, 63
Wedel, Janine, 12
Weed, Elizabeth, 104, 105
Weeks, Carly, 73, 75
Wente, Margaret, 64–5
"What's the hurry?" narrative, 60, 62, 64–6, 78. *See also* media coverage of HPV vaccine
Wiktorowicz, Mary, 98
women and girls: and COVID-19, 5; and GBA, 13, 101–2; and HPV vaccine, 8, 18–19; and HPV vaccine marketing, 6, 11, 19, 80–1, 82–3, 89–90; and HPV vaccine policymaking, 11, 92, 95–7; and media coverage, 61, 62, 63, 65–6, 67, 75, 78; medicine and othering

of, 87–9; and mothering, 36–7; and risk, 8–9, 11, 20, 84, 87, 109; and sexual health, 16, 51; and sexuality, 32–4, 48; and STI stigma, 54; and subjectivities, 17, 22–3; theoretical framework, 13–14, 17–18. *See also* gender and gendering discourses; mothering and mothers' narratives; university-aged women
"Wonder Drug's Dark Side, A," 75–6
World Health Organization (WHO), 3
Wyndham-West, Michelle, 98

Yukon, 108

Zaloom, Caitlin, 10, 17–18, 111–12
Zilber, Tamar, 14–15
zur Hausen, Harald, 6, 69, 109

www.ingramcontent.com/pod-product-compliance
Ingram Content Group UK Ltd.
Pitfield, Milton Keynes, MK11 3LW, UK
UKHW011550280525
458906UK00006B/20/J